Essentials of Pulmonary Lobectomy

Edited by Güntuğ Batıhan

Published in London, United Kingdom

Essentials of Pulmonary Lobectomy
http://dx.doi.org/10.5772/intechopen.100965
Edited by Güntuğ Batıhan

Contributors
Alberto de Hoyos, Raghav Chandra, Xiaojun Du, Jian Li, Xu Zhu, Jianglun Li, Jian Zhang, Kaiying Wang, Naveen Yadav, Sankalp Purwar, Elisabeth T. Tracy, Steven W. Thornton, Güntuğ Batıhan, Balasubramanian Venkitaraman, Lei Jiang, Suhaildeen Kajamohideen

First published in London, United Kingdom, 2023 by IntechOpen
IntechOpen is the global imprint of INTECHOPEN LIMITED, registered in England and Wales, registration number: 11086078, 5 Princes Gate Court, London, SW7 2QJ, United Kingdom

British Library Cataloguing-in-Publication Data
A catalogue record for this book is available from the British Library

Additional hard and PDF copies can be obtained from orders@intechopen.com

Essentials of Pulmonary Lobectomy
Edited by Güntuğ Batıhan
p. cm.
Print ISBN 978-1-80355-570-6
Online ISBN 978-1-80355-571-3
eBook (PDF) ISBN 978-1-80355-572-0

Meet the editor

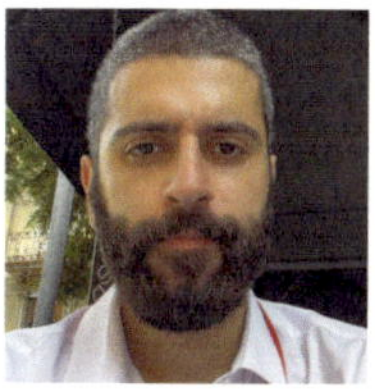

Dr. Güntuğ Batıhan is a Chief Surgeon at Kars State Hospital Thoracic Surgery Clinic in Turkey. He has made significant contributions to the literature in the field of thoracic surgery with many original research articles, international papers and book chapters. He is an editor and reviewer for several prestigious journals. His areas of interest are video-assisted thoracic surgery, minimally invasive surgery, lung cancer, esophageal cancer, mediastinal diseases and interventional bronchology.

Contents

Preface

The thoracic cavity and intrathoracic organs have remained a mystery until relatively recently because their diseases are usually fatal, and they contain fascinating but also feared pathologies in which only the most experienced surgeons are brave enough to intervene. Cumulative increases in medical and surgical knowledge, transferred over generations, have enabled thoracic surgeons gradually to widen the scope of surgically treatable diseases.

Pulmonary lobectomy, which is the subject of this book, has undergone changes in terms of surgical technique and indications over time and still continues to do so. Today, with the help of technological developments, we are able to achieve larger surgery with smaller incisions, which is every surgeon's ideal. The minimally invasive thoracic surgery approach, which started with simple pleural-parenchymal interventions, has now reached a level where advanced lung resections from a single incision are successfully performed. We are now able to push the limits of minimal invasiveness with awake/tubeless VATS approaches, which have become increasingly popular in recent years, and it is certain that we will be even more successful in this regard in the future.

Unfortunately, the number of open-access textbooks in such an important area is limited. The difficulty of accessing a resource that deals with the theoretical and practical foundations of pulmonary lobectomy in an organized manner, blended with current literature knowledge, has been the driving force in the creation of this book.

I am proud to present this book, in which leading authors on pulmonary lobectomy are contributing significantly to the pool of scientific knowledge in this important field, and which will provide a basic resource for trainee and specialist physicians interested in the field of thoracic surgery. The book covers surgical anatomy of the lung, thoracoscopic and robotic lobectomy, lobectomy in the pediatric age, and post-lobectomy intensive care.

Güntuğ Batıhan
Department of Thoracic Surgery,
Kars Harakani State Hospital,
Kars, Turkey

Section 1

Surgical Anatomy

Chapter 1

Surgical Anatomy of the Lungs

Güntuğ Batıhan

Abstract

Anatomical lung resections are specialized procedures that require a good knowledge of anatomy and high surgical experience. Individual isolation and dissection of hilar structures, including pulmonary arteries, pulmonary veins, and bronchus, are the basic steps of anatomic lung resection. Today, lobectomy is still the gold standard treatment method in many lung pathologies, especially in early-stage lung cancer. In-depth knowledge of anatomy, including variations, is required to perform this surgical procedure safely and successfully, which has a relatively high risk of intraoperative complications. Technological developments and the spread of minimally invasive surgery paved the way for the recording of procedures and their use for educational purposes and that ushered in a new era in surgical education. These developments in video-assisted surgery, which is an excellent advantage for patient comfort and education, have made the digital exploration of the surgeon impossible and increased the importance of theoretical anatomy knowledge even more. This chapter will discuss the lobar distribution of the lung, tracheobronchial airway, vascular structures, and their variations.

Keywords: anatomy, lobectomy, surgery, variations, video-assisted thoracic surgery

1. Introduction

Historically, the first lung resections were based on mass ligation of the hilum [1–3]. With the development of anesthesia techniques and increasing surgical experience, anatomical resections of the lung are performed with the isolation and transection of artery, vein, and bronchial structures separately. This makes the hilar anatomy of the lung and its possible variations important. In this chapter, it is planned to discuss the anatomy of the lung from the perspective of the thoracic surgeon, accompanied by intraoperative figures (**Figures 1–3**).

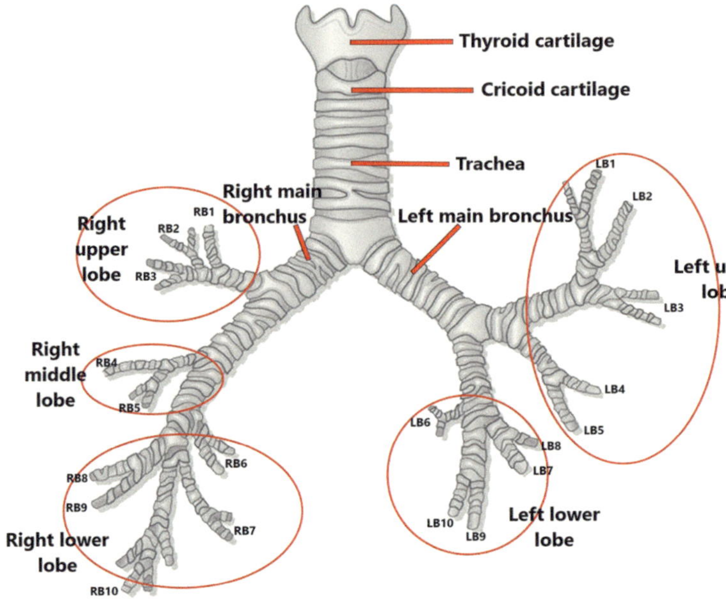

Figure 1.
Tracheobronchial anatomy (Boyden's nomenclature). Right side: RB1: Apical bronchus, RB2: Anterior bronchus, RB3: Posterior bronchus, RB4: Lateral bronchus, RB5: Medial bronchus, RB6: Superior bronchus, RB7: Medial basal bronchus, RB8: Anterior basal bronchus, RB9: Lateral basal bronchus, and RB10: Posterior basal bronchus. Left side: LB1: Apical bronchus, LB2: Posterior bronchus (LB1 + LB2 forms apicoposterior bronchus), LB3: Anterior bronchus, LB4: Superior lingular bronchus, LB5: Inferior lingular bronchus, LB6: Superior bronchus, LB7 + LB8: Anterior basal bronchus, LB9: Lateral basal bronchus, and LB10: Posterior basal bronchus.

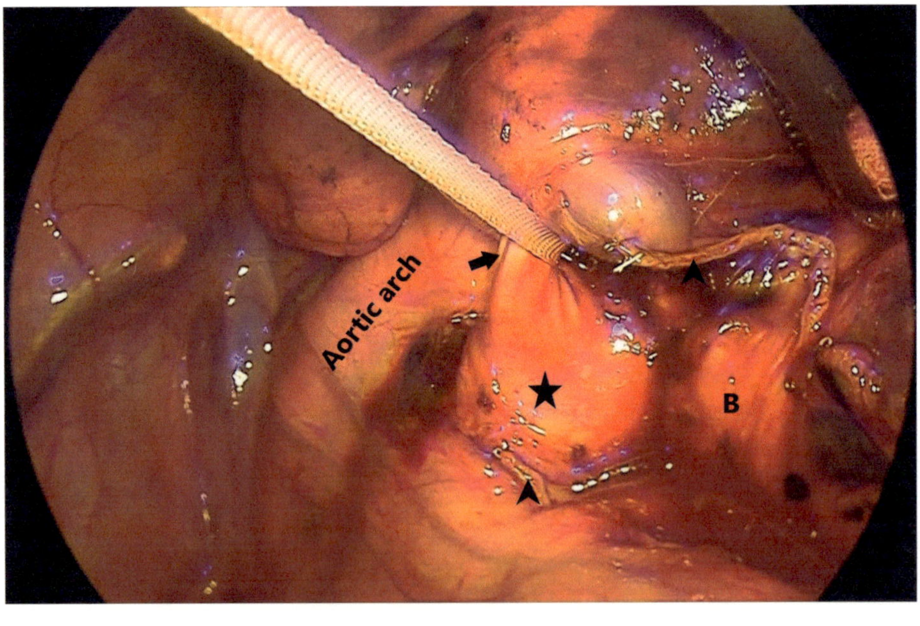

Figure 2.
After the transection of the left superior pulmonary vein, the pulmonary artery and its first branch are clearly observed. Asterisk indicates the left main pulmonary artery. The arrow indicates the apicoposterior segment artery. "B" indicates the left main bronchus. Triangles indicate proximal and distal parts of the upper lobe vein stump.

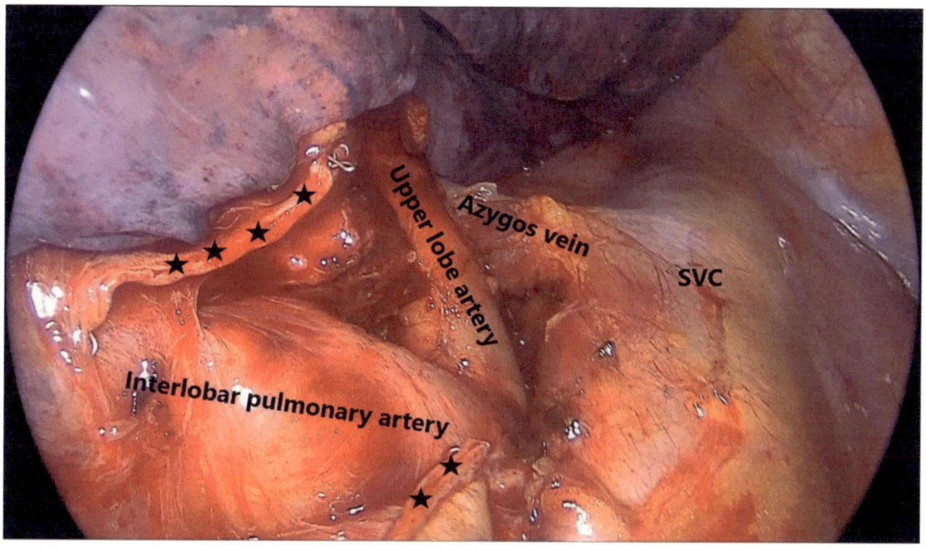

Figure 3.
After the transection of the right superior pulmonary vein, the upper lobe pulmonary artery and interlobar artery are clearly observed. Asterisks indicate proximal and distal parts of the upper lobe vein stump. SVC: superior vena cava.

2. Tracheobronchial tree

The tracheobronchial tree transmits air from the upper respiratory tract to the lung parenchyma. The right and left bronchial systems contain some differences.

The left main bronchus is longer than the right main bronchus. The left upper lobe bronchus arises from the anterosuperior of the main bronchus and divides into two, forming the upper and lower bronchial divisions. The upper division divides

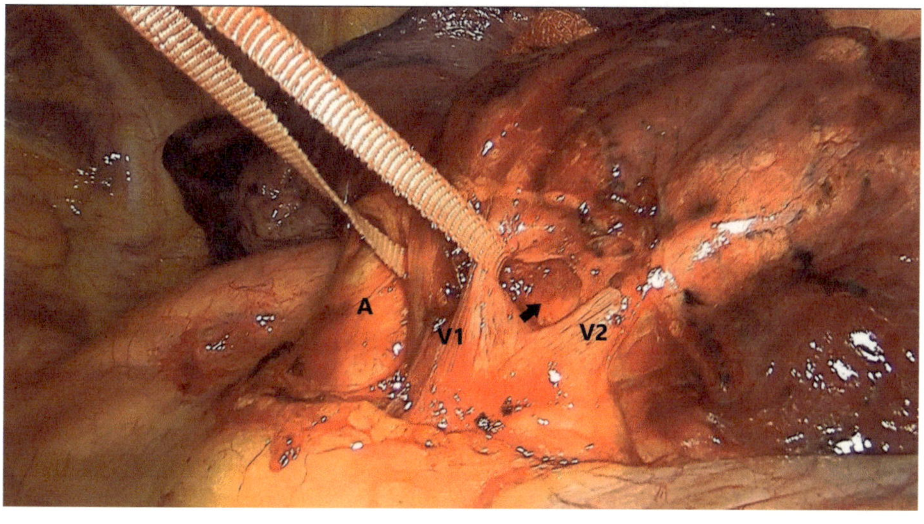

Figure 4.
The left upper lobe tri-segment vein (V1) was dissected and retracted with a silicone vessel loop. A: left main pulmonary artery. V2: lingular vein. Arrow indicates the left main bronchus.

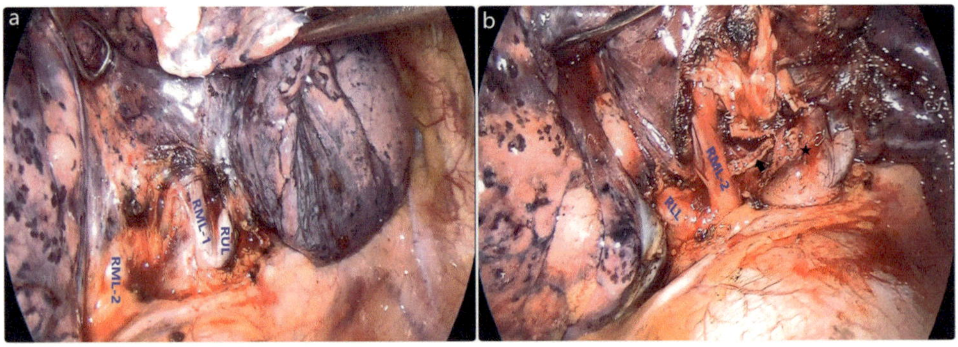

Figure 5.
The variation of the middle lobe vein is observed in a case who underwent a middle lobectomy. The middle lobe is drained by two vein branches that drain into the superior (RML-1) and inferior (RML-2) pulmonary veins. Arrow indicates transected middle lobe bronchus. Asterisk indicates transected RML-1.

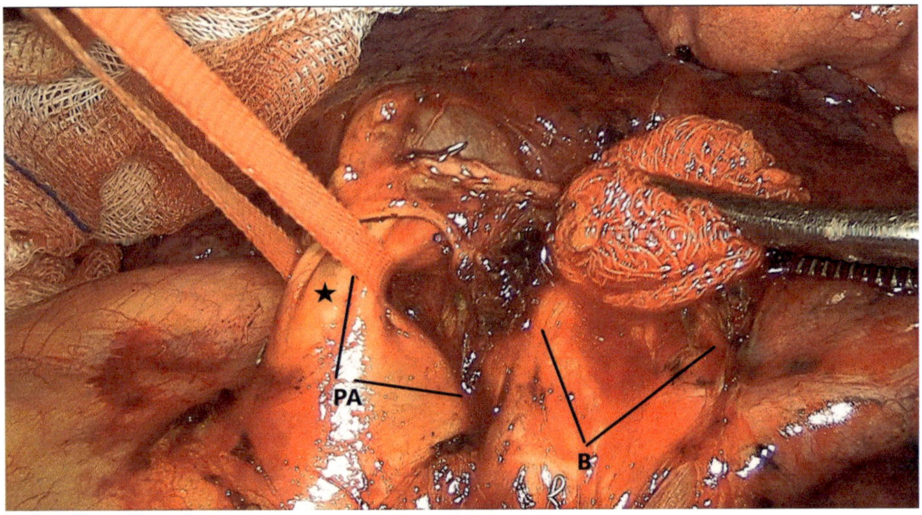

Figure 6.
View of the left hilum after transection of the superior pulmonary vein. PA: pulmonary artery. Asterisk indicates the apicoposterior artery. B: left main bronchus. The lines indicate the bifurcations of the pulmonary artery and bronchus.

into two to form the apical-posterior and anterior segmental bronchi. The lower division, also known as the lingular bronchus, divides into the superior and inferior lingular segments. The lower lobe bronchus is relatively short due to the branching of the superior segment bronchus. There may be differences in the nomenclature of the basal segments on the left side. The anterior and medial basal segments of the left lower lobe branch from the same root. For this reason, some authors state that there are four basal segments in the left lower lobe (**Figures 4–6**) [4–7].

Unlike the left upper lobe bronchus, the right upper lobe segment bronchi branch separately as apical, posterior, and anterior. Middle lobe bronchus originates from the lateral wall of the intermediate bronchus and bifurcates into medial and lateral segment bronchi. After the superior segment bronchus is arise, a total of five basal segment bronchi branch separately.

3. Pulmonary artery

3.1 Left pulmonary artery

After originating from the heart, the pulmonary artery courses in the posterior and superior direction and divides into the left and right main pulmonary arteries below the aortic arch. The left pulmonary artery is located above and slightly anterior to the left main bronchus. It curves behind the upper lobe bronchus and enters the interlobar fissure. The first branch is usually the apicoposterior segment artery. The anterior segment artery usually arises in the interlobar fissure. Although it is rare, the apical, posterior, and anterior segment arteries can be branched separately. There are two common variations in the anterior artery. First, the anterior segment artery branches close to the hilum as the first branch of the pulmonary artery. The second variation is that it arises as a branch of the lingula artery within the interlobar fissure. The lingula segment artery usually branches at the level of the lower lobe superior artery. Basal segment arteries are localized parallel to the corresponding segmental bronchi (**Figures 7–9**).

It should be noted that variations of the left upper lobe artery are very common, and the left upper lobe artery can give 2–7 branches, therefore the surgeon should always be alert for possible variations [8, 9].

3.2 Right pulmonary artery

The right pulmonary artery lies anterior and posterior to the upper lobe bronchus and gives a single root branch just before entering the interlobar fissure. This branch

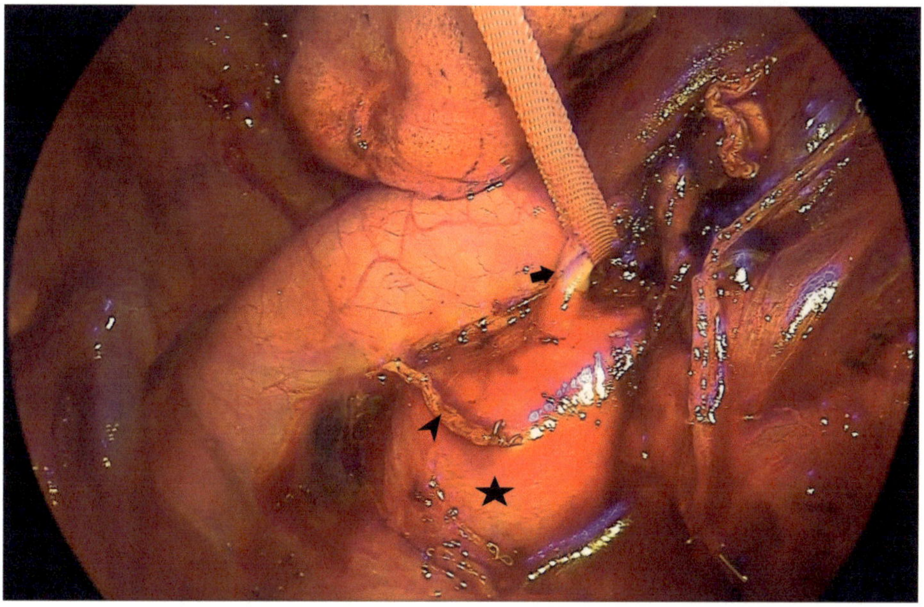

Figure 7.
The anterior segment artery (arrow) seen after the transection of the apicoposterior artery (triangle) was dissected and retracted with a silicone vessel loop. Asterisk indicates the left main pulmonary artery.

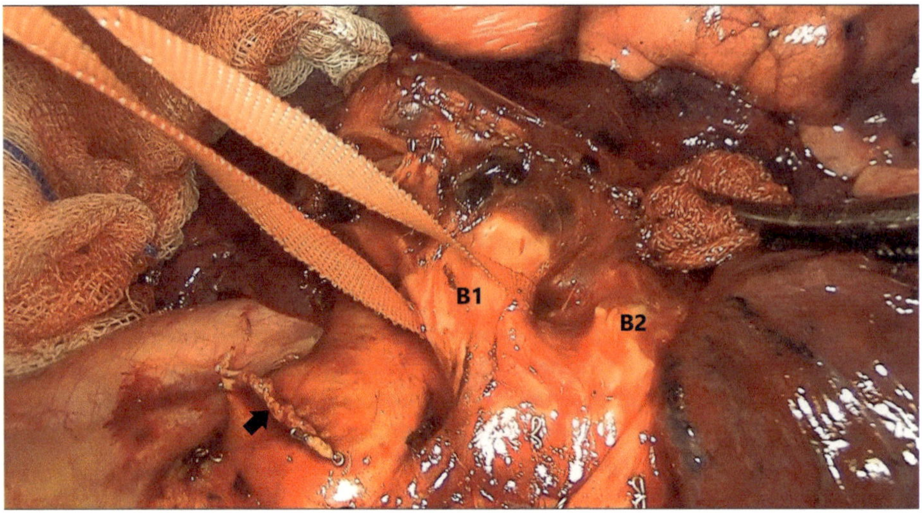

Figure 8.
View of the left hilum after transection of the upper lobe vein and apicoposterior artery. Arrow indicates the stump of the apicoposterior artery. B1: upper lobe tri-segment bronchus. B2: lingular bronchus.

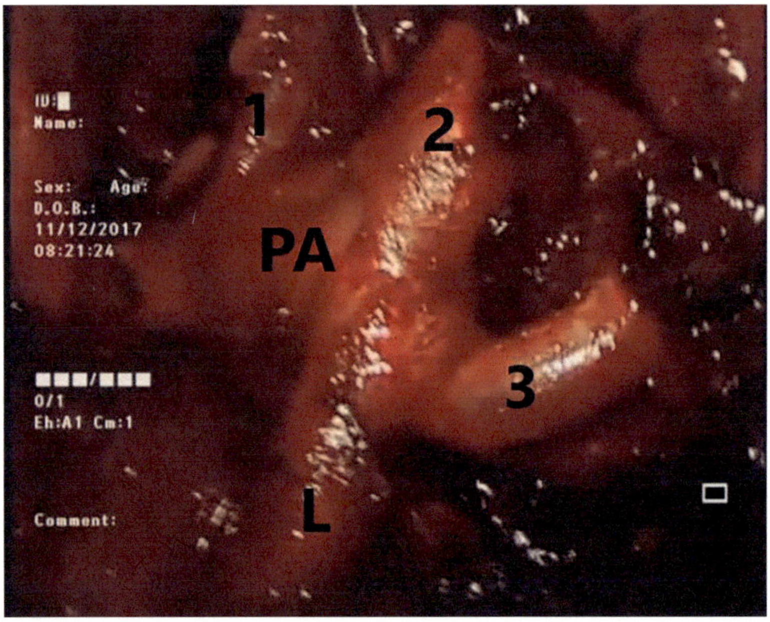

Figure 9.
The placement of the left pulmonary artery and its branches in the interlobar fissure. PA: pulmonary artery. L: lingular artery. 1 + 2: lower lobe superior segment arteries. 3: basal segment artery.

divides into the apical and anterior segment arteries. These branches supply most of the upper lobe. The posterior ascending artery feeding the posterior segment arises deep within the interlobar fissure (**Figure 10**).

Variations of the right upper lobe artery are common. Apical and anterior branches may arise separately. The posterior ascending artery may arise from the

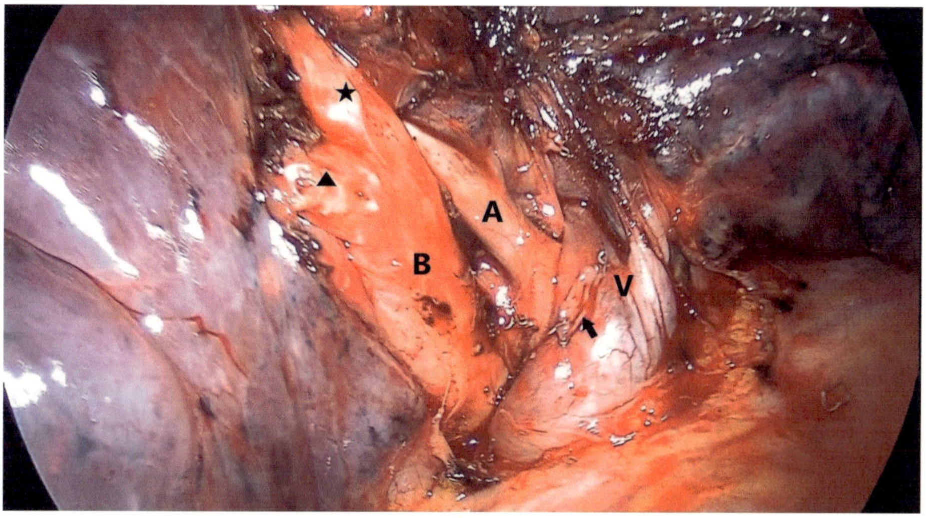

Figure 10.
The appearance of the right hilum after transection of the middle lobe vein. A: interlobar pulmonary artery. V: upper lobe vein. B: bronchus intermedius. The arrow indicates the stump of the middle lobe vein. Asterisk indicates the middle lobe bronchus. The triangle indicates the lower lobe bronchus.

middle lobe artery or the lower lobe superior segment artery. In 10% of the patients, the posterior ascending artery may be absent.

The middle lobe artery arises from the junction of the horizontal and oblique fissures and divides into two branches, medial and lateral. Sometimes a third accessory middle lobe branch can be seen.

The superior segment artery arises at the level of the middle lobe artery and divides into two branches. These branches may arise separately in some cases. In total, four basal segment arteries arise close to the lung parenchyma [8–10].

4. Pulmonary vein

4.1 Left pulmonary vein

The left pulmonary vein is the most anterior structure of the left lung hilum. The names of the segment veins of the upper lobe are similar to the names of the bronchi, as apicoposterior, anterior, and ligula.

The inferior pulmonary vein lies inferior and posterior to the superior pulmonary vein. It is located between the pleural folds, superior to the pulmonary ligament. It is best seen posteriorly. It consists of lower lobe superior and basal segment veins [8, 9, 11].

4.2 Right pulmonary vein

The right superior pulmonary vein is located anterior and slightly inferior to the right main pulmonary artery. It consists of the apical anterior, posterior, and middle lobe veins, from top to bottom, respectively. Cases where the middle lobe vein drains only into the inferior pulmonary vein or into both the superior and inferior pulmonary veins have been reported.

The inferior pulmonary vein is located below and posterior to the superior pulmonary vein, and drains the entire lower lobe. On the left, it has two main branches: the lower lobe superior segment vein and the basal veins. It is best seen posteriorly with the lung retracted anteriorly.

5. Surgical anatomy of the pulmonary hilum

The surgeon must know the location of the anatomical structures in the pulmonary hilus and their proximity to each other in order to perform safe dissection.

The unsymmetrical structure and location of the heart in the sagittal plane have created some differences between the right and left pulmonary hiluses in terms of anatomical neighborhoods.

In this section, it is planned to discuss the locations of the anatomical structures in the right and left pulmonary hilum from a surgical perspective.

5.1 Left hilum

The uppermost structure in the left lung hilum is the main pulmonary artery. The main pulmonary artery lies slightly above the main bronchus and curves behind the upper lobe bronchus to enter the interlobar fissure. After transection of the superior pulmonary vein, the main bronchus and the bifurcation of the lobe bronchi can be seen.

It should be kept in mind that the esophagus located medially and posteriorly may be injured during the dissection of the left main bronchus, especially in cases with severe adhesions between the mediastinal structures.

The inferior pulmonary vein is located superior to the pulmonary ligament, between the pleural folds. On the left side, the distance of the inferior pulmonary vein outside the pericardium is usually very short. This may lead to the unintended opening of the pericardium during dissection.

In some cases, the upper and lower pulmonary veins merge outside the pericardium and enter the pericardium as a single root [12, 13].

5.2 Right hilum

The most cephalic structure in the right hilum is the main bronchus. The main pulmonary artery is located anterior and inferior to the bronchus, so when the anterior approach is preferred, transection of the arterial branches leading to the upper lobe is required for visualization of the upper lobe bronchus.

After the main pulmonary artery gives apical and anterior branches, the posterior segment artery branches within the interlobar fissure.

However, this pulmonary artery branch, named posterior ascending artery, is not observed in the interlobar fissure in approximately 10% of the cases [14].

The middle lobe artery arises proximal to the lower lobe superior segment artery. Unlike the left lung, vein branches belonging to the posterior segment can be seen in the interlobar fissure, so this should be kept in mind when performing arterial dissection. After the posterior segment vein branches from the superior pulmonary vein, it moves posteriorly and enters the interlobar fissure. Therefore, care should be taken not to injure the posterior segment vein during the dissection or encircling of the superior pulmonary vein while performing the right upper lobectomy.

Conflict of interest

The author declares that he has no competing interests related to this chapter.

Author details

Güntuğ Batıhan
Kars Harakani State Hospital, Kars, Turkey

*Address all correspondence to: gbatihan@hotmail.com

References

[1] Kittle CF. The history of lobectomy and segmentectomy including sleeve resection. Chest Surgery Clinics of North America. 2000;**10**:105-130

[2] Lindskog GE. A history of pulmonary resection. The Yale Journal of Biology and Medicine. 1957;**30**:187-200

[3] Paget S. The Surgery of the Chest. Bristol, England: John Wright & Co.; 1896

[4] Drevet G, Conti M, Deslauriers J. Surgical anatomy of the tracheobronchial tree. Journal of Thoracic Disease. 2016;**8**(Suppl. 2):S121-S129

[5] Walker CM, Rosado-de-Christenson ML, Martínez-Jiménez S, Kunin JR, Wible BC. Bronchial arteries: Anatomy, function, hypertrophy, and anomalies. Radiographics. 2015;**35**(1):32-49

[6] Furlow PW, Mathisen DJ. Surgical anatomy of the trachea. Annals of Cardiothoracic Surgery. 2018;**7**(2):255-260

[7] Mieczkowski B, Seavey BF. Anatomy, Head and Neck, Trachea. Treasure Island (FL): StatPearls Publishing; 2021

[8] Warren WH, Milloy FJ. Pulmonary vascular system and pulmonary hilum. Thoracic Surgery Clinics. 2007;**17**:601-617

[9] Kandathil A, Chamarthy M. Pulmonary vascular anatomy & anatomical variants. Cardiovascular Diagnostic Therapy. 2018;**8**(3):201-207

[10] Elliott FM, Reid L. Some new facts about the pulmonary artery and its branching pattern. Clinical Radiology. 1965;**16**:193-198

[11] Porres DV, Morenza OP, Pallisa E, et al. Learning from the pulmonary veins. Radiographics. 2013;**33**:999-1022

[12] Guido Guerrero W, Gonzalez-Rivas D, Hernandez Arenas LA, et al. Techniques and difficulties dealing with hilar and interlobar benign lymphadenopathy in uniportal VATS. Journal of Vision Surery. 2016;**2**:23. Published 2016 Jan 31

[13] Fieira Costa E, Delgado Roel M, Paradela de la Morena M, et al. Technique of uniportal VATS major pulmonary resections. Journal of Thoracic Disease. 2014;**6**:S660-S664

[14] Gossot D, Seguin-Givelet A. Anatomical variations and pitfalls to know during thoracoscopic segmentectomies. Journal of Thoracic Disease. 2018;**10**(Suppl. 10):S1134-S1144

Section 2

Video-Assisted Thoracoscopic Surgery (VATS) Lobectomy

Chapter 2

Perspective Chapter: Essentials of Lobectomy under Video-Assisted Thoracoscopic Surgery for Non-Small-Cell Lung Cancer

Jian Li, Xu Zhu, Jianglun Li, Jian Zhang, Kaiying Wang and Xiaojun Du

Abstract

The morbidity and mortality of lung cancer rank second and first respectively in malignant solid tumors worldwide. As we all know, surgical resection is the cornerstone of comprehensive treatment of non-small-cell lung cancer (NSCLC). The current National Comprehensive Cancer Network (NCCN) guidelines for NSCLC suggest that for medically operable disease, resection is the preferred local treatment modality, anatomic pulmonary resection is preferred for the majority of patients with NSCLC, and video-assisted thoracoscopic surgery (VATS) or minimally invasive surgery should be strongly considered for patients with no anatomic or surgical contraindications. With many advantages, uniportal VATS (u-VATS) has been widely accepted and used. Therefore, in this article, we attempted to review the essentials of lobectomy under u-VATS for NSCLC.

Keywords: non-small-cell lung cancer, video-assisted thoracoscopic surgery, lobectomy, uniportal

1. Part 1. General principles

1.1 Introduction

Currently, the morbidity and mortality of lung cancer rank second and first respectively in malignant solid tumors worldwide [1, 2]. Right upper lobe has the highest incidence of lung cancer (23.8%–47.0%) among the five lung lobes [3–8]. As we all know, surgical resection is the cornerstone of comprehensive treatment of non-small-cell lung cancer (NSCLC). The current National Comprehensive Cancer Network (NCCN) guidelines for NSCLC suggest that for medically operable disease, resection is the preferred local treatment modality, anatomic pulmonary resection is preferred for the majority of patients with NSCLC, and video-assisted thoracoscopic surgery (VATS) or minimally invasive surgery (including robotic-assisted approaches) should be strongly considered for patients with no anatomic or surgical contraindications [9]. Because VATS, compared with thoracotomy, is associated with reduced length of hospital stay, less postoperative pain, fewer postoperative complications, more rapid recovery to normal life, and less pulmonary injury without compromising oncology principles [10]. Previously, VATS was conventionally performed under multiportal (m-VATS). Compared with m-VATS, uniportal VATS (u-VATS) has the advantages of direct view, easy learning, less operation time and postoperative drainage duration, decreased postoperative pain and hospitalization, diminished inflammatory response, or faster access to chemotherapy [4, 11, 12]. Consequently, u-VATS has been widely accepted and used. Therefore, in this article, we attempted to review the essentials of lobectomy under u-VATS for NSCLC.

1.2 Instrument

Due to the restricted interspace available under u-VATS, the fewer processing instruments used the better. **Figure 1** shows the instruments we commonly use. Among them, the suction with a slightly curved tip is recommended to obtain more operating space and angles. In addition, a manual-control electric hook is recommended to relieve the discomfort caused by standing on one leg when using a foot-control one too long. Furthermore, the ring forceps clamping a small gauze are used to turn and tow the lobes, instead of clamping the lobes directly, to reduce exudation from the residual lung after surgery. A high-definition thoracoscopic system is recommended too, because most of the procedures of lobectomy have to be finished very precisely. Meanwhile, a thoracoscopy with a freely rotatable optical fiber is also recommended to obtain more viewing angles. Since a three-dimensional thoracoscopic system can provide a high-definition and stereoscopic view, it is highly recommended for beginners. A 5 mm thoracoscope can further reduce the length of the incision;

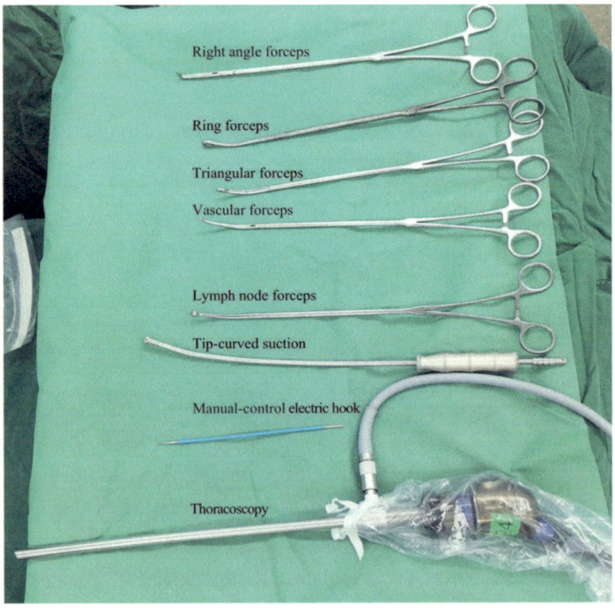

Figure 1.
The instruments commonly used.

however, the technical requirements for the surgeon and the assistant holding the thoracoscopy are harder for its smaller view. Finally, the recommended length of the staple cartridge used for vessels and bronchus is 30 mm or 45 mm, so that there is sufficient space and angle to place it into the interstice between the tissues to be cut.

1.3 Anesthesia and position

1.3.1 Anesthesia

Commonly, patients are anesthetized with intravenous coupled with inhaled anesthetics, and ventilation is maintained under contralateral endobronchial intubation with double-lumen endobronchial tube. For experienced surgical teams, tubeless anesthesia under regional combined with general anesthesia can be used.

1.3.2 Position for patient

The patient is placed in the contralateral decubitus position, and then the operating table is adjusted to a jackknife position to widen the intercostal space and elevate the hilum, which would facilitate intraoperative processing (**Figure 2**).

1.3.3 Position for surgeon and assistant

In general, the display screen is placed on the back of the patient near the head end. The surgeon stands on the upper ventral side, while the assistant stands on a low-rise foot stool on the lower ventral side. This position could increase the interspace between the thoracoscopic body and the operating instruments and could further reduce mutual interference (**Figure 3**). In order to facilitate processing, the position of the surgeon and the assistant could be exchanged when cut the lower pulmonary ligament and dissect the groups 8 and 9 lymph nodes. If there are two movable display screens and the assistant is very experienced, the assistant can stand on the back of the patient to further increase the interspace.

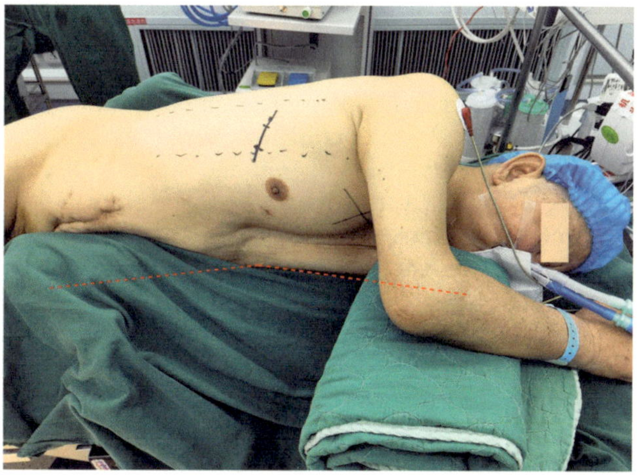

Figure 2.
The position for patient. The patient is placed in the contralateral decubitus position, and then the operating table is adjusted to a jackknife position.

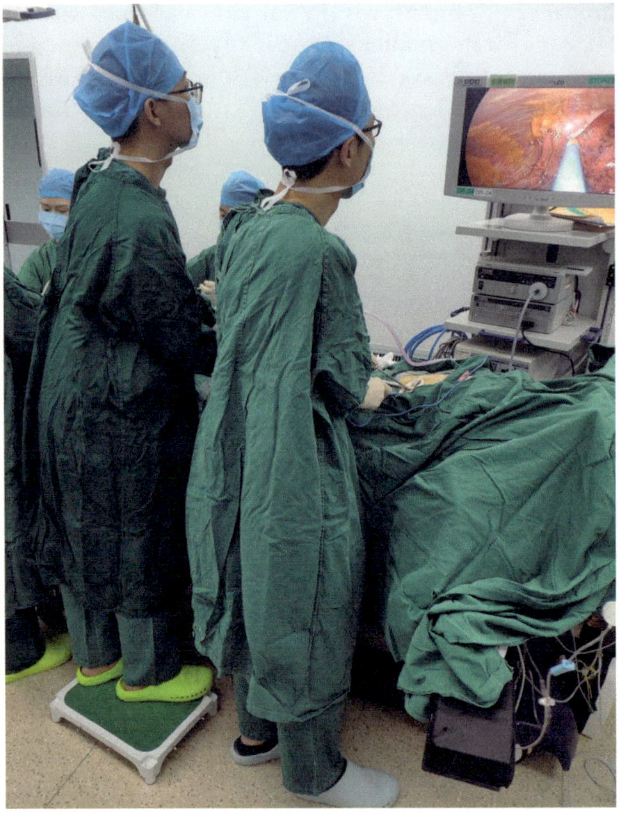

Figure 3.
Position for surgeon and assistant. The surgeon stands on the upper ventral side, while the assistant stands on a low-rise foot stool on the lower ventral side.

1.3.4 Incision and orders of placing instruments

The location of the incision is very important. It directly affects the smoothness and safety of the processing. An optimal choice of incision will make the placement of a stapler smoother under better angle. We generally make all the incision at the fifth intercostal space, except for left upper lobectomy at the fourth, from the anterior axillary to the mid-axillary line. It can not only ensure the smoothness and safety of the processing, but also facilitate the conversion to thoracotomy by lengthening the incision if necessary. Commonly, the incision is made about 3–4 cm in length. For beginners or low volume centers, the length of incision could be appropriately extended and gradually shortened after their experience is mature and stable. This can ensure the operation safe and shorten the learning curve. Incision protective cover is used to reduce staxis and facilitate the entry and exit of instruments. The orders of placing the thoracoscopy and instruments are as follows: the thoracoscopy is always close to the upper border of the incision and fixed with a string or an infusion tube to reduce the fatigue of the assistant. When the lobes need to be towed to expose the operating area, the ring forceps should be close to the lower edge of the thoracoscopy or the lower border of the incision to ensure sufficient operating interspace for the surgeon to avoid mutual interference. The dominant hand of the surgeon holds an energy device (such as an electric hook or an ultrasonic scalpel) with the nondominant hand holding a suction or a long forceps to enter the thoracic cavity through the lower border or middle of the incision. As for whether it is better to hold an electric hook or an ultrasonic scalpel in the dominant hand, and a suction device or a long forceps in the nondominant hand, each has its own advantages and disadvantages. It mainly depended on the experience and habits of the surgeon. However, when in the learning phase, surgeons should try to use a fixed combination mode to shorten the learning curve. The author is used to holding an electric hook in the dominant hand with a suction in the nondominant hand. Because the tip of the electric hook is smaller which can perform a finer anatomy, and because that the suction can not only suck the smog generated by the energy device and the staxis exuded from the operating area in time to maintain a clear vision, but also can expose the operating area. Moreover, in the event of an accidental massive bleeding caused by a major vessel broken, the suction can be used to press it in time to control the bleeding and suck the blood to ensure a clear vision, which could provide a favorable condition for the next treatment (**Figure 4**).

1.3.5 Specimen extraction

The resected lobe is bagged and dragged to the incision. After removing the incision protective cover, two ring forceps are used to drag the lung tissue and pull it out. If the lesion is longer than the incision, scissors are used to cut it into small in the bag. Here, the bag is in a semi-tight state. Then, the scissors are slightly opened with either lateral border close to the inner surface of the bag and slowly interposed to cut the lesion small. It can prevent scissors from cutting through the bag. After extracting the resected lobe, intersegmental, interlobar, and/or hilar lymph nodes are removed in vitro.

1.3.6 Systemic mediastinal lymphadenectomy

The extent of systemic mediastinal lymphadenectomy on the right side includes groups 2R, 3A, 3P, 4R, 7, 8, and 9 and groups 3A, 4 L, 5, 6, 7, 8, and 9 on the left. En bloc resection is used to ensure complete resection and reduce small residues. That is, the lymph nodes and pericentral adipose tissue are completely removed with the

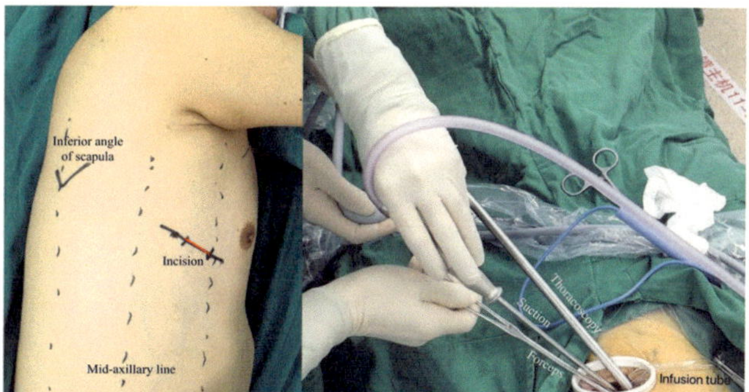

Figure 4.
Incision and orders of placing instruments. Left, the incision is made at the fifth intercostal space from the anterior axillary to the mid-axillary line. Right, the orders of placing the thoracoscopy and instruments.

surrounding normal tissue as the boundary. It is relatively difficult to remove the lymph nodes of groups 2, 4, and 7. It is recommended to completely split the mediastinal pleura and use the surrounding normal tissue as the boundary to dissect to the depths layer by layer, rather than tunneling to the depths at one point. This can facilitate the exposure of the view and process. An ultrasonic scalpel can be used to reduce the difficulty of lymph node resection, because it can not only reduce bleeding, but also achieve the functions of dissecting, pulling, and cutting simultaneously, which thereby reduce the use and replacement of other instruments.

When resect group 2 and 4 lymph nodes, a suction (or other instrument) is used to push the azygos vein up, and ultrasonic scalpel is used to dissect lymph nodes and pericentral adipose tissue with the anterior edge of the trachea, the surface of the pericardium, and the posterior edge of the superior vena cava as the boundary. Then, the mediastinal pleura is split along the superior border of the azygos arch, the posterior border of the superior vena cava, and the anterior border of the trachea in a "△" pattern. After the whole piece of lymph nodes and pericentral adipose tissue being pushed posteriorly and upwardly with suction (or other instrument),

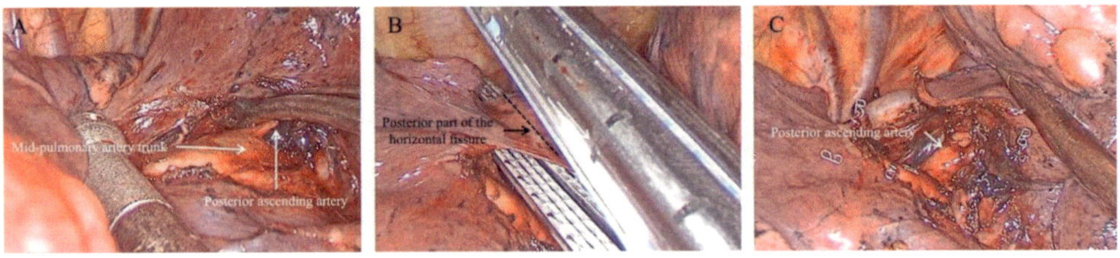

Figure 5.
Cut the posterior horizontal fissure with tunnel technique. A. Tunneling the fissure. B. Stapling the fissure. C. The outcomes after posterior horizontal fissure being cut off.

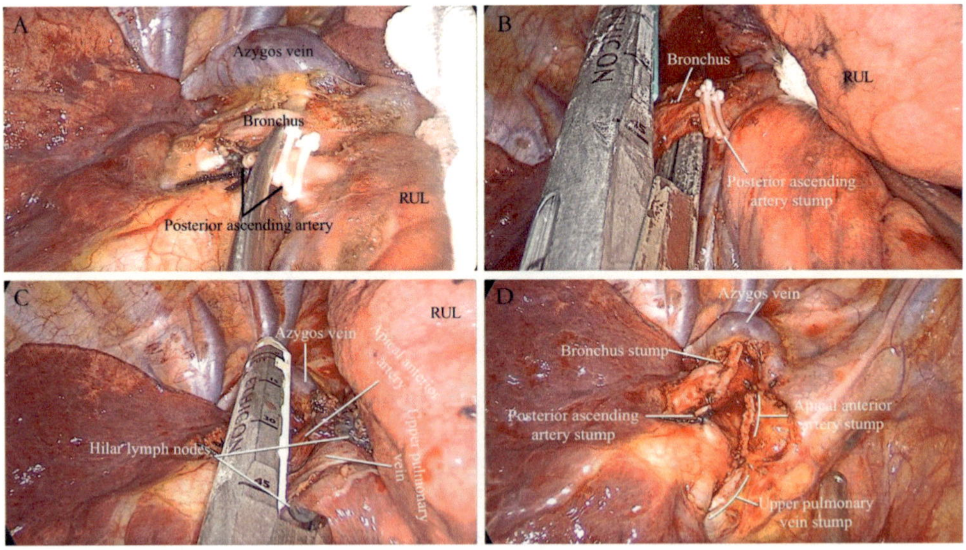

Figure 6.
The procedure of "From posterior inferior to anterior superior." A. Cutting the posterior ascending artery. B. Cutting the right upper bronchus. C. Cutting the remaining upper vessels simultaneously. D. The outcomes after right upper lobe being removed.

ultrasonic scalpel is used to dissect them cephalad gradually until being completely removed. Care should be taken when dissecting is performed near the junction of the vagus nerve and the brachiocephalic artery on right side or arch of aorta on left side, since the recurrent laryngeal nerves come from there. Blunt and sharp dissection is used interchangeably before the vagus nerve and the recurrent laryngeal nerve being clearly identified to avoid nerve damage (**Figure 5**).

When resect group 7 lymph nodes, the middle and lower lobs are first pulled anteriorly and inferiorly at the posterior hilum with a clamped gauze to fully expose the carina area. Then, the mediastinal pleura is split along the superior border of the inferior pulmonary vein, the posterior border of the right main bronchus, and the anterior superior border of the esophagus in a "△" pattern. Suction (or other instrument) is used to push the whole piece of lymph nodes and pericentral adipose tissue backward and upward, and then ultrasonic scalpel is used to completely remove them cephalad (**Figure 6**).

1.4 Dealing with special problems

1.4.1 Pleural adhesion

Pleural adhesion is often seen in diseases such as pleurisy, lobar pneumonia, obstructive pneumonia caused by massive or central lung cancer. In the past, pleural adhesion was considered a contraindication for VATS. But with the accumulation of experience and the improvement of instruments, thoracic surgeons now generally believe that there are more advantageous to dissect pleural adhesion with VATS for better viewing angle, finer dissection, and less bleeding. Of course, in the case of pleural adhesion caused by extensive rind thoracotomy is still recommended. Because the rind is too tough to make interspace for thoracoscopic process. After the incision is made, the adhesion around the incision is bluntly mobilized with fingers so that the thoracoscopy and processing instruments can be placed. Afterward, although the process is time-consuming and needs patience, the pleural adhesion dissecting can be completed with the cooperation of the curved suction and the electric hook. When the adhesion is close to some major vessels, it can remain and does not have to be completely removed, so as to avoid damage to the major vessels to cause massive bleeding or even threaten the patient's life.

1.4.2 Massive bleeding

Massive bleeding caused by broken vessels is a relatively common but serious accident in lobectomy and can occasionally be fatal. It is more common in pulmonary artery injury and rupture, while veins are less likely to rupture due to its good elasticity. It is more common in central lung cancer, lymph node calcification, neoadjuvant radiotherapy, and/or chemotherapy. In such cases, preparations for thoracotomy should be done before surgery and finer dissecting is needed during surgery. Especially when turning and pulling the lobes, it should be gentle to avoid tearing the root of the vessels. When vessel is broken and bleeding, the surgeon should keep calm. First, use suction or gauze to compress the proximal end of the broken vessel to stop bleeding. When suction is used, the location and size of the rupture can be directly observed. Then, the surgeon should decide the next treatment strategy based on the location, size of the rupture, and his or her experience, such as repair with suture, hemo-lock clamp, conversion to thoracotomy, or pulmonary artery trunk blocking, etc. The treatment suggestions are as follows:

Location	Vessel sate	Size	
		≤5 mm	>5 mm
Branch	Bound	Keep dissecting	Repair with suture or conversion to thoracotomy
	Unbound	Hemo-lock clamp	Hemo-lock clamp or repair with suture
Trunk	Bound	Repair with suture	Conversion to thoracotomy
	Unbound	Repair with suture	Conversion to thoracotomy or pulmonary artery trunk blocking

1.4.3 Difficult hilum

It refers to the situation that the hilar tissue is difficult to dissect due to the unclear and tough boundary for various reasons. It is more common in central lung cancer, lymph node calcification, neoadjuvant radiotherapy, and (or) after chemotherapy. Faced with such a situation, the surgeon should fully evaluate its resectability before surgery based on CT scan and experience. During operation, surgeon should not persist in a constant order or method of resection, but should treat it flexibly. If intraoperative exploration estimates that thoracoscopic resection is difficult, it should be timely and forwardly converted to thoracotomy, or directly thoracotomy after preoperative evaluation. Generally, it is recommended to deal with the relatively easily resectable tissue first to provide an opportunity for the more difficult one. Sometimes, it might be useful to lower the level of difficulty by splitting the pericardium and then cutting the pulmonary vein off or blocking the pulmonary artery trunk. In addition, for calcified lymph nodes, since it is the pericentral tissue that metastasizes, while itself (especially when it is completely calcified) hardly metastasizes, it is reasonable to resect it partially rather than completely. If the lateral wall of the artery trunk (<1/3 circumference) is invaded or cannot be unbound, a tri-stapler can be used to remove part of the lateral wall and the lesion simultaneously to ensure the safety of the process.

1.5 Conversion to thoracotomy

Although lobectomy under u-VATS has many advantages, thoracotomy is still better from the perspective of surgical safety. Therefore, in order to ensure the safety of patients, under any circumstance, if the surgeon is not fully confident to proceed with the next process or an uncontrollable event has occurred, it must be immediately converted to thoracotomy without hesitation. According to the emergency state when converting, it is divided into planned and forced conversion to thoracotomy. The former is that the surgeon forwardly decides to convert to thoracotomy when he or she estimates that the next process cannot be performed very safely based on their experience. At this time, the condition is relaxed and operations can be performed in an orderly manner. Generally, the anterolateral incision is lengthened to about 10 cm or through which the surgeon can reach the chest cavity with one hand for auxiliary process. Forced conversion to thoracotomy is an emergency that has occurred beyond the capability of the surgeon to handle under u-VATS. In order to save the patient's life, it has to be converted to thoracotomy immediately. It is generally seen in massive bleeding caused by major vessels broken. At this moment, the condition is very tense. The surgeon has to race against time to control the bleeding. According to the state of bleeding, the chest wall can be incised layer by layer or just once.

1.6 Drainage tube placement and incision suture

At the end of the surgery, another incision is usually made to place drainage tube. However, we could place it at the same incision to minimize invasiveness [13]. First, when the u-VATS was completed, the skin and subcutaneous tissue were pulled up and the intercostal muscle in the same intercostal space was transpierced with a mosquito forceps about 2.0 cm beyond the distal end of the incision site. Second, the drainage tube was clamped and punctured into the cavity, which is as alike as the procedure of doing a chest drainage that is familiar to thoracic surgeons in general. Third, after the drainage tube was placed properly, the subcutaneous tissue was sutured conventionally. Fourth, the drainage tube was anchored about 1.0 cm beyond the incision with a silk thread, which was passed through the subcutaneous suture. Finally, the skin incision was closed by subcutaneous continuous suture with a 3-0 self-retaining suture (Quill TM knotless tissue-closure device, Angiotech Puerto Rico Inc., Vancouver, Canada), which was cut flush to the skin lastly. When removing, one end of the anchoring silk thread was snipped and the drainage tube was pulled out, which just like removing the stiches, and the wound was sealed with Vaseline gauze immediately.

1.7 Technological difficulty

1. U-VATS has higher requirements on assistants. The assistants need to be familiar with the surgeons' habits and to ensure the processing area clearly and sufficient extrathoracic operating space for surgeon by flexibly rotating the angle of thoracoscopic body.

2. Placement of stapler under u-VATS. Compared with multi-portal VATS, the angle is relatively limited when the stapler is placed under u-VATS. Therefore, surgeons need to completely dissect the target organ and its surroundings first and then adjust the relative position of the lobe to achieve a better angle for stapler placement. In addition, a shorter or curved-tip stapler is usually useful to reduce the difficulty of stapler placement.

2. Part 2. Right upper lobectomy under u-VATS

2.1 Different orders of hilar cut

Although some studies have shown that cutting pulmonary vein first might reduce the incidence of recurrence and prolong the survival time [14–18]. However, other studies have claimed that there is no difference in the risk of recurrence and survival time between cutting the pulmonary vein first or later [19–21]. Moreover, the first intraoperative priority is to ensure the safety of the patient and the operation. Therefore, there is no need to subject to a fixed order of hilar cut. The optimal order of hilar cut is only determined by the specific situation during the operation and the surgeon's habits. The general principle is to deal with the simple tissue first and then the more difficult ones. The common orders of hilar cut are as follows:

2.1.1 Vein-artery-bronchus (VAB)

That is, the right upper pulmonary vein is cut off first, then the branches of the artery, and finally, the bronchus. It derives from the experience of thoracotomy and theoretically minimizes the possibility of hematogenous tumor spread. In addition, when the bronchus is cut off last, the likelihood of massive bleeding, which is caused by tearing the vessels, is minimized. The main process is as follows:

1. To dissect the right upper pulmonary vein, the right upper lobe is pulled backward and caudalward to expose the anterior upper hilum. Since the right upper pulmonary vein is relatively located anteriorly and inferiorly to the hilum and is very close to the incision, it will increase the difficulty of the processing due to the poor angle and the possibility of damaging the apical anterior artery when using a stapler to cut it first. It would be more difficult due to the cover of the middle pulmonary vein if the anterior part of the horizontal fissure is incomplete. In the face of such circumstances, the following methods can be used: 1) using a tip-curved stapler; 2) ligation of the vein using sutures; 3) dissecting the distal end of the pulmonary vein and cut them off respectively; 4) dissecting the apical anterior artery and the upper pulmonary vein, then cutting them simultaneously to obtain an appropriate angle for the entry of the stapler; 5) using the "tunnel technique" (see the section of "from posterior inferior to anterior superior") to cut off the horizontal fissure first to increase the mobility of the upper pulmonary veins; 6) transferring to the following other orders of hilar cut.

2. To dissect the apical anterior artery, the right upper lobe is pulled backward and caudalward to expose the anterior upper hilum as before. The apical anterior artery is no longer covered and is easy to be exposed and cut after the superior pulmonary vein having been cut off. However, it should be noted that the apical anterior artery is located at the highest position of the hilum, so it received the greatest strength when pulling the right upper lobe backward and caudalward. Therefore, it should be as gentle as possible to avoid tearing the root of the apical anterior artery. The author encountered such a situation. It is troublesome and risky to manage once it is torn here for the short of the right upper pulmonary artery trunk.

3. Continue to pull the right upper lobe backward and caudalward to expose the anterior upper hilum, and then resect the surrounding tissue along the surface of the pulmonary artery trunk. If the lymph node does not affect the process, its proximal end is resected and pushed to the distal end of the pulmonary tissue, which will be removed in vitro after the lobectomy is completed and removed to shorten the surgical and anesthesia time. Otherwise, it should be removed first to facilitate subsequent process. Here, there might be one to two variant arterial branches occasionally, which are generally tiny. For such tiny arterial branches, suture ligation, hemo-lock clip followed by scissors or ultrasonic scalpel is recommended to use. Because when cutting them off with a stapler, it is not only easy to tear them due to poor angle but also might bleed for being too tiny.

4. If the horizontal fissure is incomplete, the right upper lobe is pulled backward and caudalward to expose the anterior upper hilum as before, and the surrounding tissue along the surface of the pulmonary artery trunk is dissected. After identifying the middle pulmonary artery branch and the posterior ascending artery branch, the incomplete horizontal fissure was cut off use the "tunneling technique" (see the section of "from posterior inferior to anterior superior") along the surface of the pulmonary artery trunk between them.

5. Then the right upper lobe is pulled forward and upward to expose the posterior lower hilum. If the horizontal fissure is complete or an incomplete one is cut off as step [4], the posterior ascending branch is no longer covered and easy to be exposed and cut off.

6. Then the right upper lobe is pulled upward to expose the hilum. The tissue around the bronchus of the right upper lobe and the proximal end of the lymph node are resected and pushed to the distal end of the pulmonary tissue. Finally, the right upper bronchus is cut off with a stapler, and the resection of the right upper lobe is completed.

2.1.2 From anterior superior to posterior inferior

That is, the apical anterior artery of the right upper pulmonary artery is cut off first, followed by the pulmonary vein and arterial variant branches, then the bronchus, and finally, the posterior ascending branch and the incomplete horizontal fissure. This order is particularly useful when the horizontal fissure is incomplete. Since the right upper lobe is always pulled backward and downward throughout the operation, the lungs are mostly prevented from turning. The main process is as follows:

1. The right upper lobe is pulled backward and caudalward to expose the anterior upper hilum. The apical anterior artery is dissected and cut off with stapler. When dissecting the apical anterior artery, its inferior border is covered by the superior border of the upper pulmonary vein. Therefore, the mediastinal pleura should be split along the superior border of the upper pulmonary vein, which is then pushed caudalward with a suction (or other device) to expose the inferior border of the apical anterior artery for safe dissection.

2. After the apical anterior artery being cut off, unless the incision is made too cephalad, the right upper pulmonary vein can be dissected and cut off relatively smoothly. When inserting the stapler, the staple cartridge should be rotated toward ventral slightly to through the interspace behind the upper pulmonary vein, which might avoid the tip of the stapler damaging the lateral wall of the pulmonary artery trunk or the possible variant arterial branches.

3. If a variant arterial branch is encountered, it is recommended to use suture ligation or hemo-lock clip or ultrasonic scalpel to cut off. The proximal end of the lymph node is dissected and pushed to the distal end of the lung tissue or directly removed.

4. After that, the right upper lobe bronchus is located at the last uppermost part of the hilum. Then, it was pulled slightly upward so that the bronchus was perpendicular to the mediastinum to increase the interspace between the bronchus and the posterior ascending artery. The tissue around the bronchi and the proximal lymph nodes are dissected and pushed to the distal end of the lung tissue or directly removed. The right upper lobe bronchus was cut off with a stapler.

5. The proximal end of the interlobar lymph nodes is dissected and then pushed to the distal end of the lung tissue or directly removed. If the posterior ascending

artery is thick (> 3 mm in diameter), it needs to be dissected and cut off separately. Otherwise, it can be stapled with the incomplete fissure using a 60 mm stapler to complete the right upper lobe resection.

2.1.3 From posterior inferior to anterior superior

That is, the posterior ascending artery is first cut off, then the bronchus, and finally, the upper pulmonary vein and the apical anterior artery (including possible variant arterial branches) are cut off simultaneously. It is especially useful when the horizontal fissure is complete. Since most of the procedure is performed with the upper lobe in its natural collapsed status, it is rarely needed to turn it over. The main process is as follows as we reported before [22]:

1. If the horizontal fissure is complete, only the visceral pleura at the horizontal fissure need to be split with an energy device. If not, the "tunnel technique" is used to cut it off. First, the upper lobe is pulled backward and upward using a suction (or other instrument) to expose the anterior hilum, and the mediastinal pleura is split along the upper border of the middle pulmonary vein. Second, the proximal end of the adipose tissue and lymph nodes is dissected and pushed to the distal end of the lung tissue or directly removed until the surface of mid-pulmonary artery trunk is exposed. After that, forceps or ultrasonic scalpel is used to bluntly and sharply dissect the tissues along the

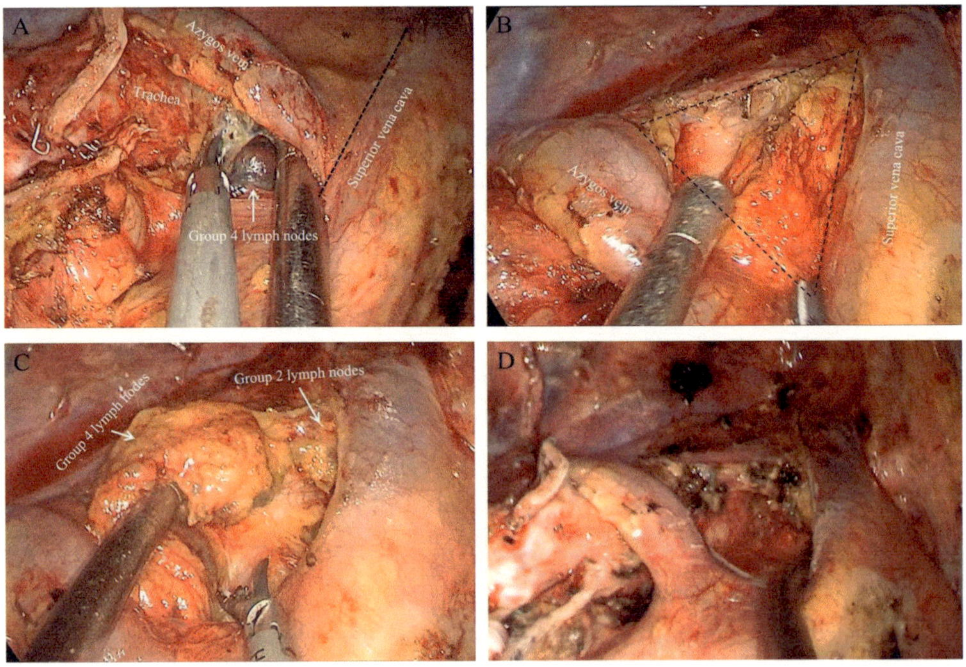

Figure 7.
Resecting group 2 and 4 lymph nodes. A. a suction is used to push the azygos vein up, and ultrasonic scalpel is used to dissect lymph nodes. B. The mediastinal pleura is split in a "△" pattern. C. The whole piece of lymph nodes and pericentral adipose tissue being pushed posteriorly and upwardly with suction. D. The outcomes after group 4 and 2 lymph nodes being removed.

surface of the mid-pulmonary artery trunk to make a factitious tunnel. Then, the anterior part of the horizontal fissure was cut off with a stapler through the factitious tunnel (**Figure 7**). After carefully identifying the posterior ascending artery, a stapler is used again to cut the posterior part of the horizontal fissure (**Figure 8**).

2. When the horizontal fissure is split, the posterior ascending branch is located at the lowest part of the right upper hilum. Then, the posterior ascending branch was dissected and cut off easily (**Figure 5**).

3. After the posterior ascending artery being cut off, there is usually a lymph node at the lower border of the upper bronchus, which is then dissected and pushed to the distal end of the lung tissue. When the anterior and superior borders of the upper bronchus are dissecting, more attention should be paid to observe whether there is dense adhesion between the apical anterior artery and the bronchus. If so, it would be treated as a difficult hilum (see the section of dealing with special problems). If not, it could be dissected along the anterior border of the upper bronchus with forceps or ultrasonic scalpel bluntly and sharply. Here, this process is relatively safe due to the lymph node separating the instrument from the anterior apical artery. Then, the right upper bronchus is cut off with a stapler.

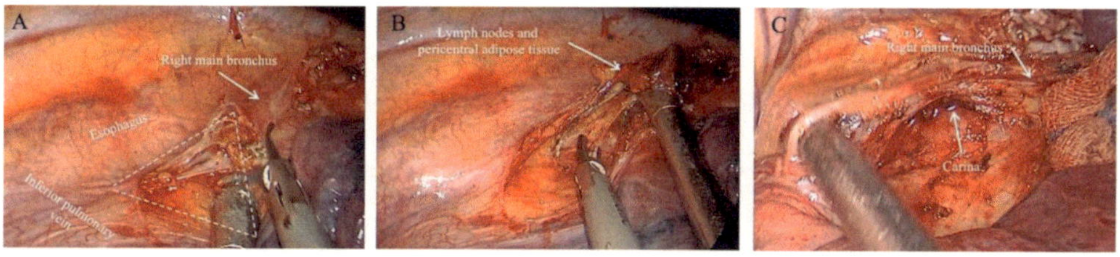

Figure 8.
A. The mediastinal pleura is split in a "△" pattern. B. The group 7 lymph nodes and pericentral adipose tissue is pushed backward and upward. C. The outcomes after group 7 lymph nodes being removed.

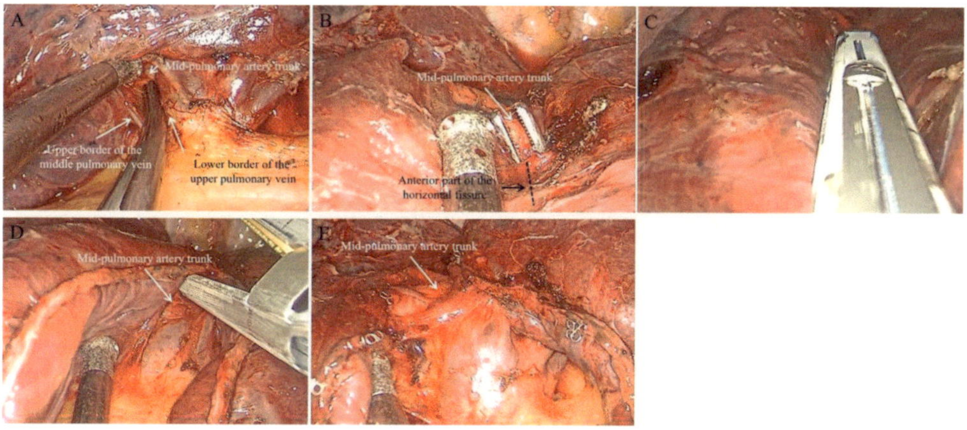

Figure 9.
Cut the anterior horizontal fissure with tunnel technique. A. To expose the mid-pulmonary artery trunk. B. Tunneling the fissure. C and D. Stapling the fissure. E. The outcomes after anterior horizontal fissure being cut off.

4. After that, the adipose tissue and the proximal end of the lymph nodes are dissected and then pushed to the distal end of the lung tissue or directly removed. If the lymph nodes are covered by possible variant arteries, it can be dissect along the surface of the pericardium posteriorly. Then the right upper lobe is pulled backward and caudalward to continue to dissect the lymph nodes anteriorly. Subsequently, the lymph nodes are pushed to the distal end of the lung tissue or removed directly. Now, the remaining upper pulmonary vessels (including the right upper pulmonary vein, the apical anterior artery, and possible arterial variant arteries) are hollowed out. And, then they are cut off simultaneously with a stapler. Finally, the right upper lobe is completely removed (**Figure 9**).

3. Part 3. Right middle lobectomy under u-VATS

Right middle lobectomy under u-VATS is relatively easy for its hilum is superficial to the mediastinum, especially when the fissures are complete.

1. First, the right upper and middle lobes are pulled backward and upward to expose the anterior hilum. The mediastinal pleura is split along the inferior border of the upper and middle pulmonary vein. And the middle pulmonary vein is then dissected and cut off with stapler. It is comparatively easy, because the backward of the middle pulmonary vein is the middle bronchus, which is less likely to be injured.

2. If the horizontal fissure is incomplete, the "tunnel technique" is used to cut it off as described before. Then, the medial segmental artery is clearly visible, which comes from the inferior of the middle-pulmonary artery. It is dissected and cut off with stapler or hemo-lock clip or ultrasonic scalpel.

3. The proximal end of the oblique fissure is split with ultrasonic scalpel or electric hook to expose the lateral segmental artery, which is then dissected and cut off with stapler or hemo-lock clip or ultrasonic scalpel.

4. The right middle lobe is pulled upward, and the right middle bronchus is dissected with surrounding lymph nodes and adipose tissue being dissected and pushed to the distal end of the lung tissue or directly removed. Next, the middle bronchus is cut off with stapler.

5. Finally, the incomplete oblique fissure is stapled to complete the right middle lobectomy.

4. Part 4. Right lower lobectomy with single-direction under u-VATS

The advantage of lobectomy with single directional is that the whole procedure starts from the shallowest structure of the hilum, proceeds in one direction, and cuts the fissure. This procedure is particularly useful when the oblique fissure is incomplete.

4.1 Surgical procedure

After the right lower lobe is pulled backward and cephalad, the inferior pulmonary ligament is cut to the lower boundary of the lower pulmonary vein with electric hook (**Figure 1**). And the group 8 lymph node is dissected and pushed to the distal end of the lung tissue or directly removed.

Dissect the inferior pulmonary vein and remove group 9 lymph node or push it to the distal end of the lung tissue, then separate and expand the interspace between the vein and lower bronchus by forceps (**Figure 2**).

Cut the inferior pulmonary vein off with stapler (**Figure 3**).

Dissect the lower bronchus and separate it from the lower pulmonary artery with a forceps by close to the upper boundary of the lower bronchus to avoid injuring the artery (**Figure 4**). Then cut the lower bronchus off with stapler (**Figure 7**).

Remove group 11 lymph node or push it to the distal end of the lung tissue. Then dissect the lower pulmonary artery and suspend it with suture (**Figure 8**).

Cut off the lower lobe artery with stapler (**Figure 9**).

Finally, cut off the oblique fissure with stapler to finish the right lower lobectomy (**Figure 5**).

4.2 Essential technology for right lower lobectomy with single direction under u-VATS

The sheath of the inferior pulmonary vein, especially the surrounding pleura, must be completely split to facilitate the placement of stapler. Moreover, the middle pulmonary vein may sometimes drain into the inferior pulmonary vein, so it needs to be carefully identified during dissecting.

More attention should be paid when separating lower bronchus to avoid injuring vessels. There are often lymph nodes around the bronchus. Sometimes these lymph nodes closely adhere to the bronchus and vessels, making it difficult to separate the interspace between the bronchus and vessels. On this occasion, it is impossible to place the stapler due to insufficient space. Therefore, the lower lobe bronchus should be cut off with scissors and then suture the bronchial stump after removing the lobe. In addition, it should be noted that the dissecting of the upper boundary of the lower bronchus should be performed on the interior of the middle lobe bronchus, because the lower lobe is pushed upward. Otherwise, if the dissecting is too close to the mediastinum, the middle bronchus may be injured or cut accidentally. Furthermore, the lower bronchus should be cut off at an appropriate distance (about 5 mm) to the middle lobe bronchus to avoid the stenosis of the middle lobe bronchus and subsequently postoperative atelectasis or occurrence of bronchopleural fistula.

In most cases, the lower pulmonary artery trunk can be cut off with one stapler. If the dorsal segment artery is far from the basal artery trunk, they need to be cut off respectively. In addition, when dissecting the artery, it should be gentle to avoid massive bleeding caused by tearing it.

5. Part 5. Left lower lobectomy under u-VATS

Left lower lobectomy under u-VATS can be performed as similar as right lower lobectomy reported before. Here, we describe another procedure, which is more commonly used.

1. First, the left lower lobe is pulled backward and cephalad to expose the inferior hilum. The inferior pulmonary ligament is cut to the lower boundary of the lower pul-

monary vein with electric hook or ultrasonic scalpel. And the group 8 lymph node is dissected and pushed to the distal end of the lung tissue or directly removed.

2. If the oblique fissure is incomplete, the "tunnel technique" is used to cut it off as described before. Then, the basal artery trunk and the dorsal segment artery are clearly visible. If they are close to each other, they can be cut off with one stapler. Otherwise, they should be cut off respectively.

3. The left lower lobe is pulled upward, and the bronchus is dissected with surrounding lymph nodes and adipose tissue being dissected and pushed to the distal end of the lung tissue or directly removed. Finally, the bronchus is cut off with stapler to complete the left lower lobectomy.

6. Part 6. Left upper lobectomy under u-VATS

Left upper lobectomy under u-VATS is comparatively difficult for its special hilar anatomy and more frequent variant artery. Comparing with the right hilum, the left hilum is cephalad higher, and most of the arteries of the left upper division are covered by the upper bronchus. Therefore, the incision is made at the fourth intercostal space to facilitate dissection and placement of stapler.

1. First, the left upper lobe is pulled backward and caudalward to expose the anterior hilum. The mediastinal pleura is split along the upper hilum. A long right-angle forceps or an auricular appendage forceps is used to dissociate the upper vein from the upper bronchus and pulmonary artery trunk to make an artificial tunnel. When making the tunnel, the tip of the forceps should be rotated toward ventral slightly to through the interspace behind the upper pulmonary vein. It might avoid damaging the lateral wall of the pulmonary artery trunk. The tunnel should be made as wide as possible to facilitate the placement of the stapler. Otherwise, a tip-curved stapler is needed to cut the vein off.

2. Then, the left upper lobe is pulled toward ventral and caudal to expose the posterior hilum. The posterior mediastinal pleura is split, and the anterior and apicoposterior segmental arteries are dissected along the pulmonary artery trunk. After that, the anterior segmental artery is stapled with the upper lobe being pulled backward and caudalward again.

3. The left upper lobe is pulled toward ventral and caudal to expose the posterior hilum once again. And the apicoposterior and lateral subsegmental arteries are cut off respectively. Here, the apical and posterior subsegmental arteries might come from the pulmonary artery trunk respectively. They can be cut off simultaneously if they are close to each other or respectively if not. The lateral subsegmental artery is usually tiny and could be cut off with hemo-lock clip or ultrasonic scalpel.

4. The left upper lobe is pulled upward, and the bronchus is dissected with surrounding lymph nodes and adipose tissue being dissected and pushed to the

distal end of the lung tissue or directly removed. Then, the bronchus is cut off with stapler.

5. The proximal end of the interlobar lymph nodes is dissected and then pushed to the distal end of the lung tissue or directly removed. If the lingular segmental artery is thick (> 3 mm in diameter), it needs to be dissected and cut off separately. Otherwise, it can be stapled with the incomplete fissure using a 60 mm stapler to complete the left upper lobectomy.

Sometimes, it is difficult to cut the pulmonary vein first because of insufficient angle for stapler placement (**Figure 6A**) or dense adhesion caused by calcified lymph node. In this case, the abovementioned procedure is reversed (**Figures 6B–F** and **10**).

1. First, the anterior part of the oblique fissure is cut off with "tunnel technique" (**Figure 6B**).

2. The lingular segmental artery is dissected and cut off (**Figure 6C**).

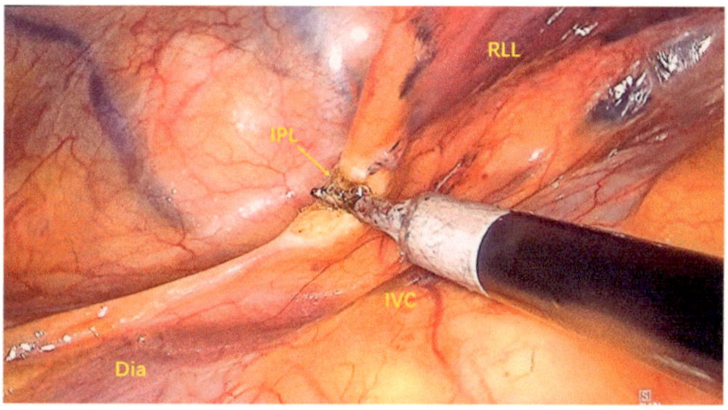

Figure 10.
Dissecting the inferior pulmonary ligament. IPL, inferior pulmonary ligament. RLL, right lower lobe. Dia, diaphragm. IVC, inferior vena cava.

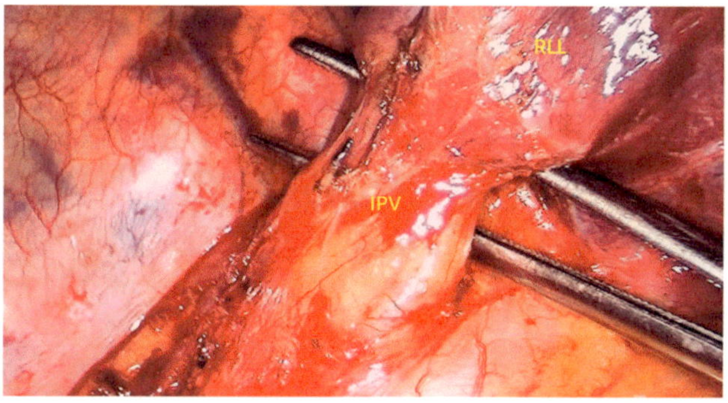

Figure 11.
Dissecting the inferior pulmonary vein. IPV, inferior pulmonary vein. RLL, right lower lobe.

3. The posterior part of the oblique fissure is cut off with "tunnel technique" (**Figure 6D**).

4. The arterial branches are dissected and cut off one by one from caudal to cephalic (**Figures 6E–F** and **10A**).

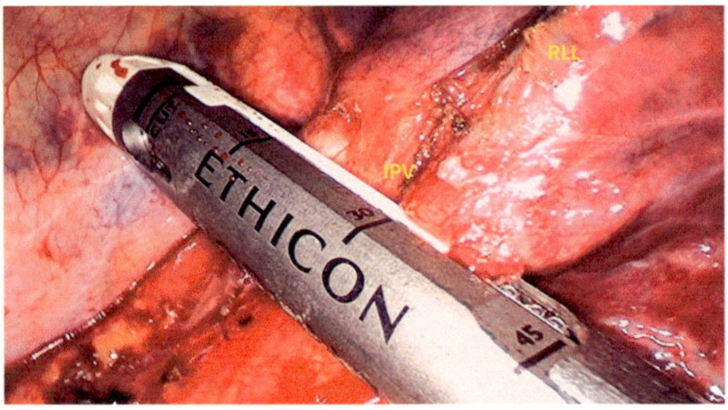

Figure 12.
Dissect the inferior pulmonary vein. IPV, inferior pulmonary vein. RLL, right lower lobe.

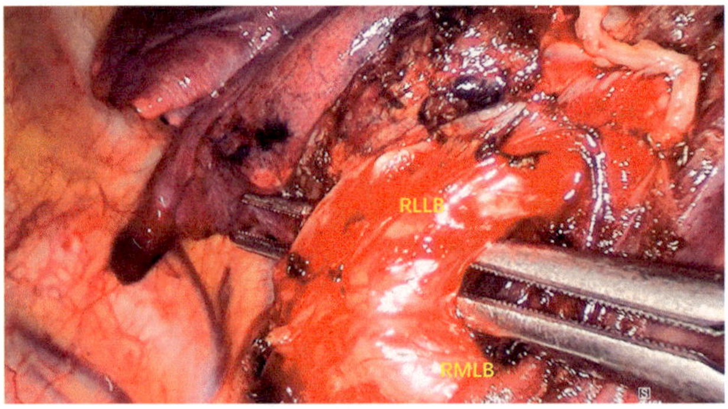

Figure 13.
Dissect the lower lobe bronchus. RLLB, right lower lobe bronchus. RMLB, right middle lobe bronchus.

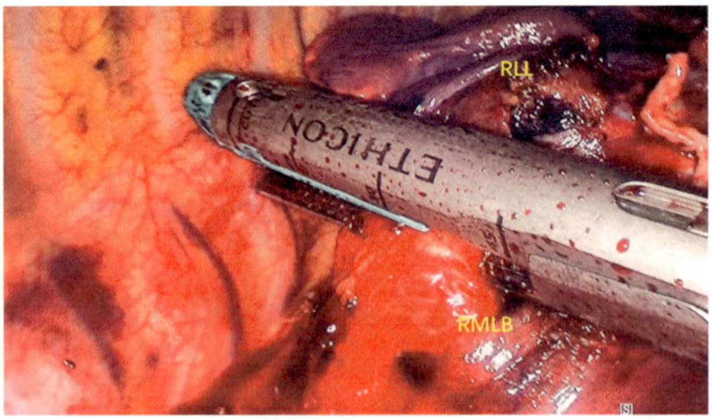

Figure 14.
Cut off the lower lobe bronchus. RLL, right lower lobe. RMLB, right middle lobe bronchus.

5. Then, the upper pulmonary vein can be cut off easily (**Figure 10B**).

6. The left upper lobe is pulled upward, and the bronchus is dissected with surrounding lymph nodes and adipose tissue being dissected and pushed to the distal end of the lung tissue (**Figure 10C**). Then, the bronchus is cut off with stapler (**Figure 10D**) to complete the left upper lobectomy (**Figures 10E** and **11–19**).

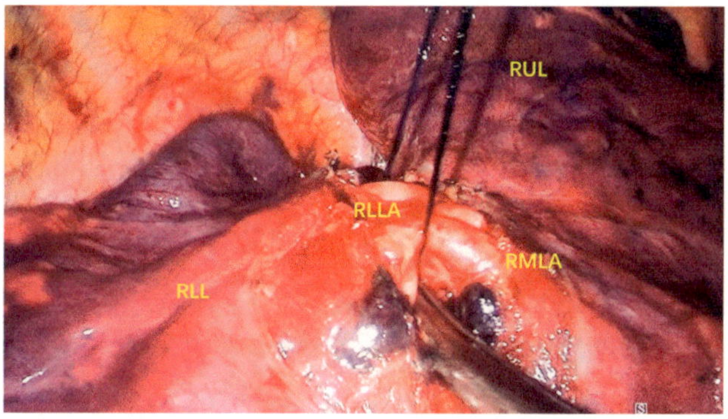

Figure 15.
Dissect the lower lobe artery. RLLA, right lower lobe artery. RMLA, right middle lobe artery. RLL, right lower lobe. RUL, right upper lobe.

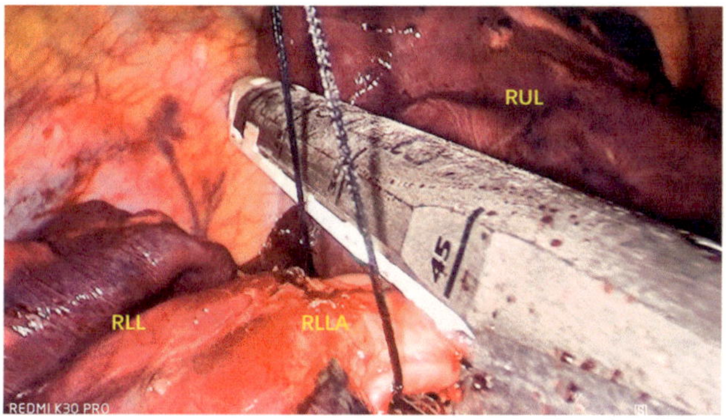

Figure 16.
Cut off the lower lobe artery. RLLA, right lower lobe artery. RLL, right lower lobe. RUL, right upper lobe.

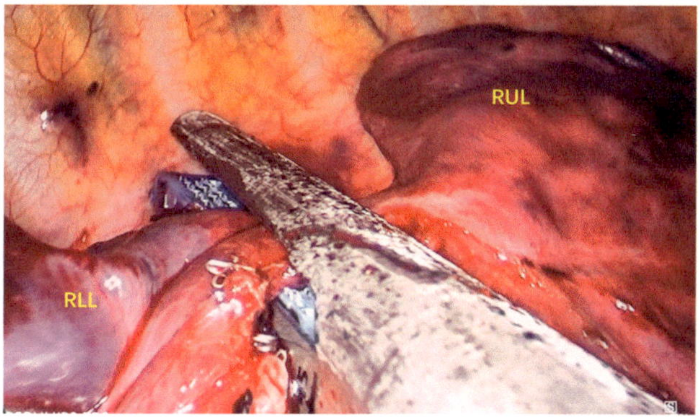

Figure 17.
Cut off the interlobar fissure. RLL, right lower lobe. RUL, right upper lobe.

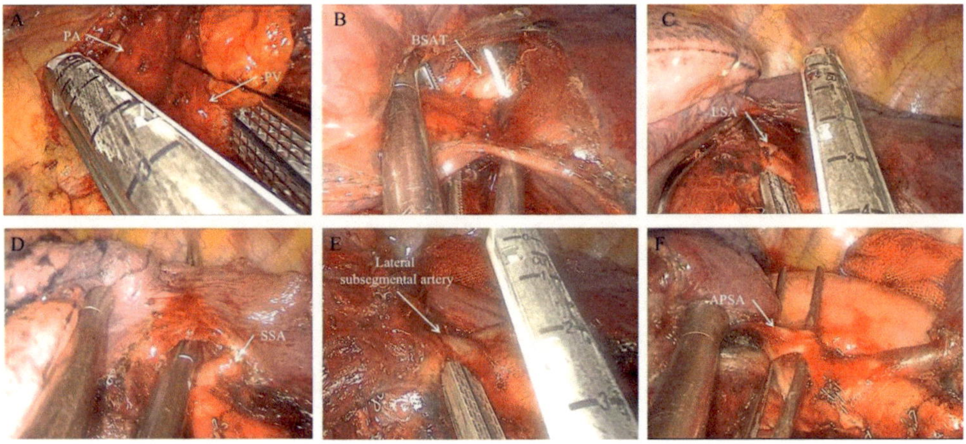

Figure 18.
The reversed procedure for left upper lobectomy. A. Insufficient angle for stapler placement. B. Dissecting the anterior part of the oblique fissure with "tunnel technique." C. Stapling the LSA. D. Dissecting the posterior part of the oblique fissure with "tunnel technique." E. Stapling the lateral subsegmental artery. F. Dissecting the APSA. PA, pulmonary artery. PV, pulmonary vein. BSAT, basal segmental artery trunk. LSA, lingular segmental artery. SSA, superior segmental artery. APSA, apicoposterior segmental artery.

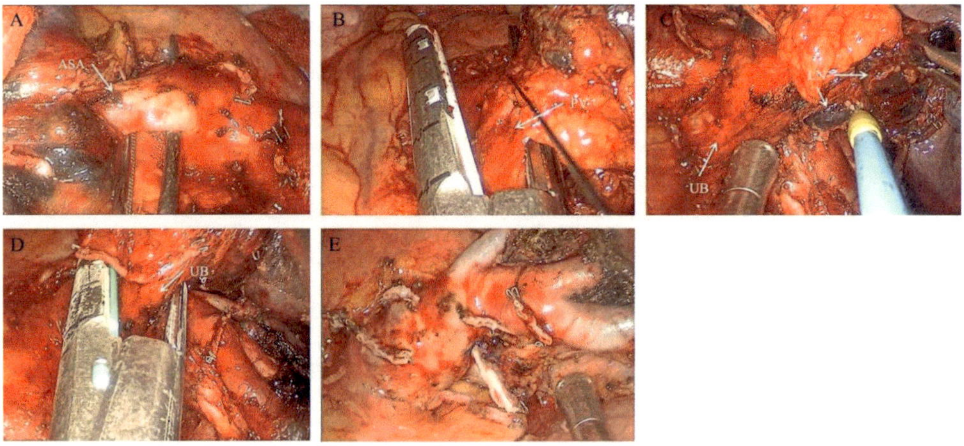

Figure 19.
The reversed procedure for left upper lobectomy (continue). A. Dissecting the ASA. B. Stapling the PV. C. The surrounding lymph nodes and adipose tissue are dissected and pushed to the distal end of the lung tissue. D. Stapling the UB. E. The outcomes after left upper lobe being removed. ASA, anterior segmental artery. PV, pulmonary vein. LN, lymph node. UB, upper bronchus.

Author details

Jian Li, Xu Zhu, Jianglun Li, Jian Zhang, Kaiying Wang and Xiaojun Du*
Department of Thoracic Surgery, The Affiliated Hospital of Guizhou Medical University, Guiyang, China

*Address all correspondence to: xj.du@foxmail.com

References

[1] Siegel RL, Miller KD, Fuchs HE, Jemal A. Cancer statistics, 2022. CA: A Cancer Journal of Clinicians. 2022;**72**:7-33. DOI: 10.3322/caac.21708

[2] Zhang S, Sun K, Zheng R, Zeng H, Wang S, Chen R, et al. Cancer incidence and mortality in China, 2015. Journal of the National Cancer Center. 2021;**1**:2-11. DOI: 10.1016/j.jncc.2020.12.001

[3] Flores RM, Park BJ, Dycoco J, Aronova A, Hirth Y, Rizk NP, et al. Lobectomy by video-assisted thoracic surgery (VATS) versus thoracotomy for lung cancer. The Journal of Thoracic and Cardiovascular Surgery. 2009;**138**:11-18. DOI: 10.1016/j.jtcvs.2009.03.030

[4] Matsuura N, Igai H, Ohsawa F, Yazawa T, Kamiyoshihara M. Uniport vs. multiport video-assisted thoracoscopic surgery for anatomical lung resection-which is less invasive? Journal of Thoracic Diseases. 2021;**13**:244-251. DOI: 10.21037/jtd-20-2759

[5] Menna C, Poggi C, Andreetti C, Maurizi G, Ciccone AM, D'Andrilli A, et al. Does the length of uniportal video-assisted thoracoscopic lobectomy affect postoperative pain? Results of a randomized controlled trial. Thoracic Cancer. 2020;**11**:1765-1772. DOI: 10.1111/1759-7714.13291

[6] Lim CG, Shin KM, Lim JS, Lim JK, Kim HJ, Kim WH, et al. Predictors of conversion to thoracotomy during video-assisted thoracoscopic surgery lobectomy in lung cancer: Additional predictive value of FDG-PET/CT in a tuberculosis endemic region. Journal of Thoracic Diseases. 2017;**9**:2427-2436. DOI: 10.21037/jtd.2017.07.40

[7] Byun CS, Lee S, Kim DJ, Lee JG, Lee CY, Jung I, et al. Analysis of unexpected conversion to thoracotomy during thoracoscopic lobectomy in lung cancer. The Annals of Thoracic Surgery. 2015;**100**:968-973. DOI: 10.1016/j.athoracsur.2015.04.032

[8] Samson P, Guitron J, Reed MF, Hanseman DJ, Starnes SL. Predictors of conversion to thoracotomy for video-assisted thoracoscopic lobectomy: A retrospective analysis and the influence of computed tomography–based calcification assessment. The Journal of Thoracic and Cardiovascular Surgery. 2013;**145**:1512-1518. DOI: 10.1016/j.jtcvs.2012.05.028

[9] Ettinger DS, Wood DE, Aisner D, Akerley W, Bauman JR, Bharat A, et al. NCCN clinical practice guidelines in oncology: Non-small cell lung cancer. Version 5. 2021. Available from: https://www.nccn.org/guidelines/guidelines-detail?category=1&id=1450. [Accessed June 16, 2021]

[10] Yao J, Chang Z, Zhu L, Fan J. Uniportal versus multiportal thoracoscopic lobectomy: Ergonomic evaluation and perioperative outcomes from a randomized and controlled trial. Medicine (Baltimore). 2020;**99**:e22719. DOI: 10.1097/MD.0000000000022719

[11] Gonzalez-Rivas D. Uniportal thoracoscopic surgery: From medical thoracoscopy to non-intubated uniportal video-assisted major pulmonary resections. Annals of Cardiothoracic Surgery. 2016;**5**:85-91. DOI: 10.21037/acs.2016.03.07

[12] Gonzalez-Rivas D, Paradela M, Fernandez R, Delgado M, Fieira E, Mendez L, et al. Uniportal video-assisted thoracoscopic lobectomy: Two years of experience. The Annals of Thoracic

Surgery. 2013;**95**:426-432. DOI: 10.1016/j.athoracsur.2012.10.070

[13] Du X, Chen G, Tian D, Xie L, Zhou H. Modified tube fixation technique for uniportal video-assisted thoracic surgery. Video-Assisted Thoracic Surgery. 2018;**3**:45-45. DOI: 10.21037/vats.2018.10.03

[14] Sawabata N, Funaki S, Hyakutake T, Shintani Y, Fujiwara A, Okumura M. Perioperative circulating tumor cells in surgical patients with non-small cell lung cancer: Does surgical manipulation dislodge cancer cells thus allowing them to pass into the peripheral blood? Surgical Today. 2016;**46**:1402-1409. DOI: 10/gnjf9k

[15] Duan X, Zhu Y, Cui Y, Yang Z, Zhou S, Han Y, et al. Circulating tumor cells in the pulmonary vein increase significantly after lobectomy: A prospective observational study. Thoracic Cancer. 2019;**10**:163-169. DOI: 10.1111/1759-7714.12925

[16] Sawabata N, Nakamura T, Kawaguchi T, Watanabe T, Ouji NS, Ito T, et al. Circulating tumor cells detected only after surgery for non-small cell lung cancer: Is it a predictor of recurrence? Journal of Thoracic Diseases. 2020;**12**:4623-4632. DOI: 10.21037/jtd-20-1636

[17] Hashimoto M, Tanaka F, Yoneda K, Takuwa T, Matsumoto S, Okumura Y, et al. Positive correlation between postoperative tumor recurrence and changes in circulating tumor cell counts in pulmonary venous blood (pvCTC) during surgical manipulation in non-small cell lung cancer. Journal of Thoracic Diseases. 2018;**10**:298-306. DOI: 10/gc845x

[18] Long X, Wu B, Zhang W, Lv G, Yu D, Peng J, et al. Effects of vessel interruption sequence during lobectomy for non-small cell lung cancer: A systematic review and meta-analysis. Frontiers in Surgery. 2021;**8**:694005. DOI: 10/gnjf9s

[19] Zhai H-R, Yang X-N, Nie Q, Liao R-Q, Dong S, Li W, et al. Different dissecting orders of the pulmonary bronchus and vessels during right upper lobectomy are associated with surgical feasibility and postoperative recovery for lung cancer patients. China Journal of Cancer. 2017;**36**:53. DOI: 10.1186/s40880-017-0220-9

[20] Kozak A, Alchimowicz J, Safranow K, Wójcik J, Kochanowski L, Kubisa B, et al. The impact of the sequence of pulmonary vessel ligation during anatomic resection for lung cancer on long-term survival – a prospective randomized trial. Advances in Medical Sciences. 2013;**58**:156-163. DOI: 10/f5bmdf

[21] Refaely Y, Sadetzki S, Chetrit A, Simansky DA, Paley M, Modan B, et al. The sequence of vessel interruption during lobectomy for non–small cell lung cancer: Is it indeed important? The Journal of Thoracic and Cardiovascular Surgery. 2003;**125**:1313-1320. DOI: 10/fm8sgq

[22] Wang K, Zhang J, Li J, Liu L, Tang Z, Du X. aBVA procedure by uniportal video-assisted thoracoscopic surgery for right upper peripheral lung cancer: A Randomized Trial. Frontiers in Oncology. 2022;**12**:828432. DOI: 10.3389/fonc.2022.828432

Chapter 3

Thoracoscopic Lobectomy in Infants and Neonates

Elisabeth T. Tracy and Steven W. Thornton

Abstract

Video-assisted thoracic surgery is a well-established approach to managing lung pathology in the adult and adolescent population. This minimally invasive strategy has also gained traction for the care of infants and neonates with congenital lung lesions. Thoracoscopic surgery for infants and neonates requires special attention to these patients' unique physiology. Careful consideration must also be given to lung isolation, the effects of insufflation, and the constraints of small working spaces. Additionally, anomalies such as congenital pulmonary airway malformations have special anatomic considerations including cystic regions and anomalous feeding vessels. However, the basic surgical principles of pulmonary resection apply to infants and children as well as adults.

Keywords: pulmonary resection, wedge resection, segmentectomy, lobectomy, thoracoscopic, video-assisted thoracic surgery, children, infants, neonates, pediatrics

1. Introduction

Thoracoscopic surgery is a minimally invasive approach to thoracic surgery wherein large intercostal incisions, rib spreading, and rib resection are avoided. Visualization for these cases depends entirely upon video monitors. There are also modified approaches to thoracoscopy where the thoracoscope is used as an adjunct to rib spreading. These approaches are known as video-assisted thoracotomy.

Minimally invasive thoracic surgery dates back to 1910 when Jacobeus treated a patient with tuberculosis by using a cystoscope to induce a therapeutic pneumothorax [1]. The field took a leap forward in 1993 with the use of thoracoscopic surgery for an anatomic lobectomy in a patient with malignancy [2]. Several large series comparing thoracoscopic surgery to open resection were completed during the early 2000s, which demonstrated feasibility, safety, and comparable outcomes—primarily in adult patients with pulmonary malignancy [3–5]. Later, Steve Rothenberg described a technique for thoracoscopic surgery in infants, which has since proved to be safe and reproducible [6, 7]. This led to the adoption of such techniques by pediatric surgeons, who now regularly make use of smaller instruments and gentle insufflation to achieve good outcomes.

Theoretical benefits to thoracoscopy include decreased postoperative pain, shorter chest tube durations, reduced length of stay, and improved cosmesis. Thus, although traditional surgical approaches such as posterolateral thoracotomy, muscle-sparing thoracotomy, trans-sternal thoracotomy, and median sternotomy remain viable options, thoracoscopy is considered the standard approach in adults when possible. A recent analysis of the Society of Thoracic Surgeons (STS) database demonstrates that thoracoscopic lobectomies account for 45% of all lobectomies performed [8]. Comparable, robust data on the prevalence of thoracoscopic approaches in infants and neonates are not available, but the approach continues to gain favor as the field of pediatric surgery advances.

2. Indications for pulmonary resection in infants and children

2.1 Congenital lung anomalies

Congenital lung anomalies are altogether uncommon, though when present they represent a common indication for surgical intervention in the infant or neonatal chest. Lesions of the lung, which are potentially amenable to surgery, include congenital pulmonary airway malformations, bronchopulmonary sequestrations, hybrid lesions, and congenital lobar emphysema. As prenatal imaging has improved, early identification of each of these lesions has increased, and the literature guiding their treatment has grown. However, specific practice guidelines are lacking, and surgeon judgment remains the driving factor in decision-making. Ultimately, the prognosis of most children with congenital lung lesions is good, and many are candidates for thoracoscopic resection as an alternative to thoracotomy.

2.1.1 Congenital pulmonary airway malformations

Congenital pulmonary airway malformations (CPAMs) are benign cystic masses of abnormal lung tissue in infants and children (**Figure 1**). They were previously referred to as congenital cystic adenomatoid malformations, or CCAMs, but the name was revised as pathologists began documenting that many of the lesions were neither cystic nor adenomatoid. Now, CPAM is an umbrella term, which includes CCAMs along with sequestrations and hybrid lesions (**Figure 2**). CPAMs are the most encountered congenital lesions of the lung. They range in severity from those that remain asymptomatic indefinitely to those that cause hydrops fetalis and fetal demise from pulmonary hypoplasia.

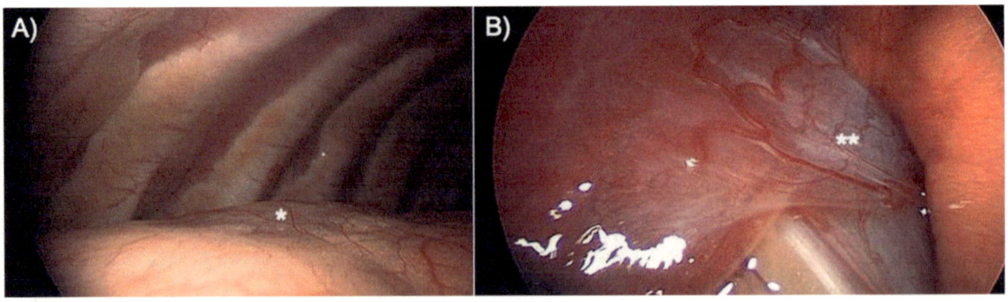

Figure 1.
A) Congenital pulmonary airway malformation (CPAM) (*) on the pleural surface B) without arterial vascular supply in the ligamentous attachment (**).

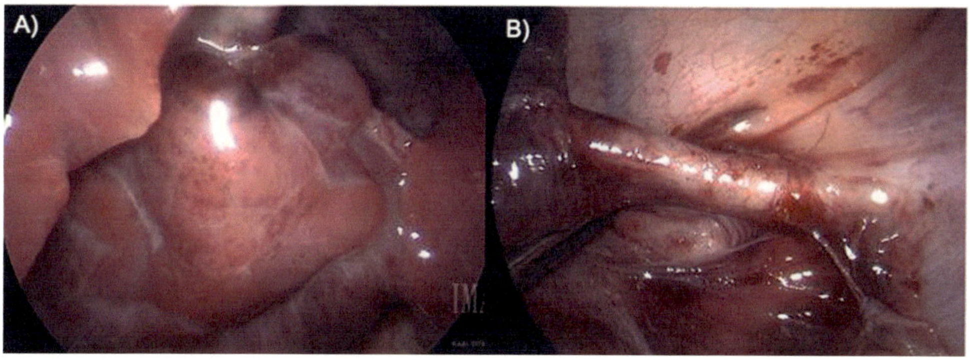

Figure 2.
A) Congenital cystic adenomatous malformation (CCAM) and B) intralobar hybrid lesion with a systemic feeding vessel.

CCAMs are most frequently classified into five groups. Type 0 lesions are exceedingly rare and typically lethal. Here the cysts arise within the trachea or bronchus [9]. Type 1 lesions are the most common, occurring in over 50% of cases, and result from the development of cystic tissue in the distal bronchus or proximal bronchiole. They can become quite large and thus may lead to the development of hydrops [10]. Type 2 lesions are found in roughly a quarter of cases and are frequently associated with congenital anomalies of other organ systems. The extent to which other organ systems are affected defines the prognosis of type 2 lesions. Type 3 lesions occur in less than 10% of cases and are believed to arise from acinar-like tissue. Type 4 lesions are found in about 10% of cases and have been associated with pleuropulmonary blastoma. These lesions are alveolar in origin [11]. Prior to birth, lesions may be classified based on cyst size. Those smaller than 5 mm are termed microcytic, whereas those larger are termed macrocytic. Microcytic lesions are associated with worse outcomes. Types 1, 2, and 4 may present as macrocytic or have elements of both. Type 3 lesions are universally microcytic [12].

CPAM size is an important predictor of outcome. The most used metric is the CPAM volume ratio, CVR. This is the ratio of CPAM/fetal head circumference, where higher ratios are correlated with hydrops fetalis and perinatal morality [13]. Although fetal hydrops is a devastating complication, most patients will be asymptomatic in the fetal and perinatal period. More commonly, patients will be asymptomatic or develop a range of symptoms including respiratory distress, pneumothorax, air leak, pneumonia, empyema, or others contributing to pulmonary abscesses. Up to 25% of initially asymptomatic lesions are expected to become symptomatic, with most of these developing around 6 or 7 months of age [14]. CPAMs may also predispose to, or conceal, malignancy, an outcome that can occur well into adulthood [15].

Symptomatic lesions necessitate surgical intervention. The management of asymptomatic CPAMs, however, is controversial and the potential for these lesions to become symptomatic or mask malignancy must be considered. The objective when operating on an asymptomatic patient is to prevent the development of functional symptoms, pneumonia, or abscess and to mitigate the risk of malignancy.

A 2017 systematic review from the American Pediatric Surgeons Association Committee on Evidence-Based Practice found extensive practice heterogeneity. Most surgeons agreed on the importance of postnatal chest X-ray and CT scan, but consensus could not be reached on optimal timing. Some advised neonatal imaging as early as 6 weeks, whereas others planned for radiographic studies between 3 and 12 months. Resection practices varied as well. Twenty-one percent advise universal resection of asymptomatic CPAMs, 24% recommend observation only for asymptomatic lesions, and the remainder make their recommendation based on lesion size, location, parental preferences, and their suspicion for malignancy [16]. It should be noted that the malignant potential of CPAMs is widely debated. Type 4 CPAMs most strongly predispose to malignancy, though the transformation potential of hybrid lesions and other CPAMs is not well defined [17]. Although there are older studies exploring this topic, the advent of improved prenatal imaging renders them obsolete as we now detected lesions that would have previously gone undetected except at autopsy. In the absence of robust practice guidelines, we favor the latter approach, where the unique presentation of each patient and surgeon judgment are prioritized.

For patients undergoing operative management, anatomic resection is the most common approach for anomalies confined to a single lobe. Early studies suggested that thoracoscopy was a safe and feasible approach that achieved comparable outcomes and shorter length of hospitalization compared with open resection [18]. More recent literature also suggests that thoracoscopic excision may reduce total complication rates [19]. It also mitigates the risk of chest wall deformity, which unlike in the adult population is a real concern for infants undergoing thoracotomy. There is evidence to support the claim the thoracoscopic approach results in less postoperative pain, fewer wound infections, and less long-term musculoskeletal sequelae [20–22]. These findings should be interpreted with caution, though, as the sample sizes are small. This is a common challenge in pediatric surgery, and ultimately, the surgeons' skill and judgment should play an important role in selecting the operative approach.

Removal of the cystic tissue allows the normal pulmonary tissue to function at capacity, and for the pathologist to obtain a definitive tissue diagnosis in patients for whom the concern for malignancy is high. It also mitigates the risk of infections in a population predisposed to recurring pneumonia. Although anatomic resection is most common, there are reports of lung sparing (LSR) resections (i.e., wedge resections or segmentectomies). The LSR approach is generally considered feasible and safe, though studies examining long-term outcomes are limited. It offers theoretical benefit over anatomic resection as the infant's alveoli continue to develop for the first 1–2 years of life [23]. As a result, lung resection during infancy is thought to be less morbid than in adults. No studies to date have examined the theoretical benefit of LSR on pulmonary function, though, and there is no evidence to suggest that the approach is superior to lobectomy for a single, asymptomatic lobar CPAM with regard to either perioperative morbidity or long-term pulmonary function [16]. We thus prefer the lobectomy for its anatomic simplicity and ensuring that the entire lesion is excised.

The optimal timing of surgery in asymptomatic patients has always been controversial. It is theoretically easier to operative in the thorax prior to the development of CPAM complications as they cause inflammatory changes, which result in a hostile operative field [24]. As a consequence, elective resection is associated with better outcomes compared with emergent surgery [25, 26]. Another important consideration for operative timing is that lung growth continues during the early childhood period. This allows for compensatory lung development after resection. So, although immediate postnatal resection is not required, there are advantages to early intervention. The single largest study examining this topic found increased morbidity associated with resection in younger than 3 months of age or less than 5 kg and increased operative time for infants older than 9 months. Thus, the authors recommended deferring elective CPAM resection until the infant was at least 3 months of age, but no older than 9 months [26].

There are also limited reports of fetal pulmonary lobectomy in fetuses with hydrops, though the significant risk of preterm labor and premature delivery must be considered. Other interventions such as pleuro-amniotic shunts can also be completed prenatally, but these operations are only offered at specialized fetal centers [16].

Given the variation in institution and surgeon practice, a robust multicenter study examining risk adjusted outcomes in CPAM patients undergoing resection would be beneficial. The overall rarity of the condition, as is often the case in pediatric surgery, makes this difficult.

2.1.2 Bronchopulmonary sequestrations

Bronchopulmonary sequestrations (BPSs) are masses of lung tissue supplied by anomalous systemic arteries, which do not participate in gas exchange as they are not connected to the tracheobronchial tree. These are the second most common type of congenital pulmonary lesion.

A BPS may be either extra- or intra-lobar depending on their relationship to functional lung tissue. Extra-lobar BPSs are fully separated from the functional lung and are surrounded by their own pleural cover. Intra-lobar BPSs are incorporated *into* the functioning lung. These lesions are compared in **Table 1**. BPSs may be identified on prenatal ultrasonography, incidentally during extra-pulmonary surgical intervention, with the development of recurrent pneumonia or abscess. There are also reports of BPS torsion presenting with sudden abdominal or chest pain necessitating immediate resection in a previously well child [27].

Like CPAMs, BPSs appear as a well-defined homogenous, echo-dense mass on prenatal ultrasonography. They can be distinguished from CPAMs by the presence of doppler flow from a systemic artery to the lesion. This finding, however, is not universally demonstrated on ultrasound, and an MRI may be necessary to distinguish between the two. CT may also be indeterminate (**Figure 3**).

Like CPAMs, the management of asymptomatic lesions remains controversial. It should be noted that intra-lobar lesions have an increased risk of developing

Characteristics	Intra-lobar sequestrations	Extra-lobar sequestrations
Proportion	75%	25%
Gender predominance	n/a	Male (3:1)
Extra-pulmonary associations	n/a	Congenital diaphragmatic hernia, vertebral deformities, and congenital heart disease
Location	Medial basal or posterior basal segment of lower left lobe	Left lobe
Diagnostic trends	May be identified prenatally, or during infancy when a child presents with recurring pneumonia or abscess.	Typically identified prenatally or as an incidental finding during surgical repair of an extra-pulmonary defect.

Table 1.
Comparison of intra- and extra-lobar pulmonary sequestrations.

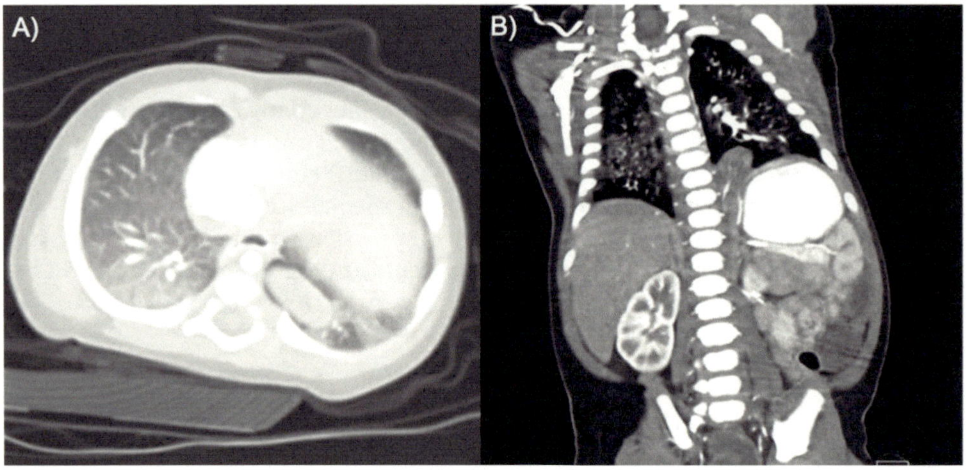

Figure 3.
A) Axial and B) coronal CT imaging of a prenatally diagnosed pulmonary lesion of unknown etiology.

symptoms, particularly those related to infection, as their connection to the functional lung tissue and the bronchopulmonary tree allows for sequestration of infectious material. Additionally, intra-lobar sequestrations are fed by arterial vessels, which most commonly arise from the abdominal aorta and may require repair of a diaphragmatic defect if traversed (**Figure 4**). These can, in some unfortunate cases, result in pulmonary overcirculation or symptomatic shunting. Both scenarios are indications for resection and preoperative embolization should be considered to mitigate intraoperative bleeding risk.

Ultimately, BPSs are monitored and managed similarly to CPAMs, with comparable variations in practice between surgeons and institutions [28, 29]. Though special attention must be paid to resection and ligation of the feeding vessels when pursuing surgery. These technical details are described in detail later in the chapter.

When surgery is performed by a surgeon well versed in thoracoscopy, outcomes with thoracoscopic surgery are comparable to thoracotomy in this population [30]. And recent evidence demonstrates the safety of this approach when applied by appropriately supervised trainees [7]. There are limited reports of a hybrid and endovascular approach to management as well, though surgical resection remains the gold standard when intervention is indicated. As prenatal imaging continues to

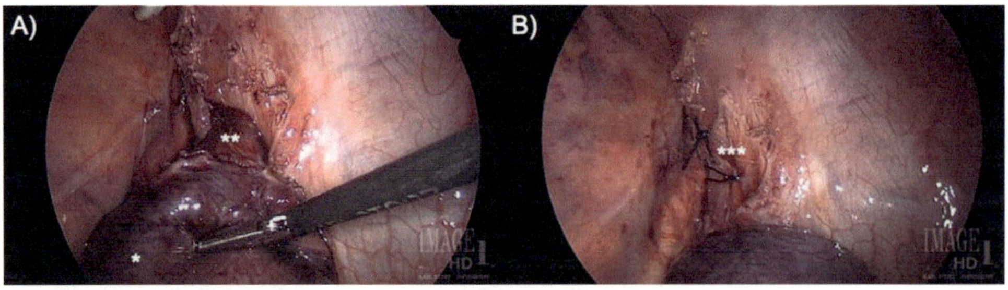

Figure 4.
A) Intralobar sequestration (*) with aortic vascularization (**) before and B) after transection with subsequent repair of diaphragmatic defect (***).

improve, rigorous practice guidelines should be developed to guide management of these increasingly diagnosed lesions.

2.1.3 Hybrid lesions

Pulmonary lesions with findings suggestive of both CPAM and BPS are possible. These are referred to as hybrid lesions, and as with the constituent defects they represent, evidence-based guidelines for management are scarce. Surgeon judgment and patient presentation are the dominant forces driving management. Consideration should be given to what has been previously described about CPAMs and BPSs.

2.1.4 Congenital lobar emphysema

Congenital lobar emphysema (CLE) is the overdistention of pulmonary tissue resulting from airway obstruction. This may affect a segment, portion of a lobe, or an entire lobe. As with the other lesions described in this chapter, CLE may be diagnosed on antenatal imaging, or be identified in the setting of a symptomatic child. Half of patients are symptomatic at birth and almost all the remainder develop symptoms within the first 6 months of life. It is uncommon to identify CLE in an asymptomatic child.

The infant with congenital lobar emphysema presents with acute, life-threatening respiratory distress. CLE has a 3:1 predominance for male infants with implication of the upper lobe being most common. Only infrequently are the lower lobes involved. Bi-lobar involvement is rare but described [31]. Chest X-ray is usually diagnostic and demonstrates hyperinflation of the involved lobe with compression of the contralateral lung and mediastinal shift [32].

Management of CLE depends on severity of presentation. Nonoperative management is recommended in patients with mild to moderate symptomatology. In the presence of severe pulmonary disfunction or ongoing clinical progression, the gold standard approach to management is a lobectomy. Transient lobar occlusion with balloon endoscopic balloon dilation has been suggested as a mechanism for evaluating the impact of surgical resection *a priori* in patients for whom surgical management is equivocal [31].

It is important to state that CLE must not be confused with a tension pneumothorax, as placement of a chest tube into the overinflated lung can be disastrous. Additionally, since the respiratory distress is of obstructive rather than restrictive etiology, intubation and positive pressure ventilation can worsen respiratory function by forcing more air into the lungs and further expanding them. Expert neonatologists and anesthesiologists should be involved in the care of these infants, who are often managed non-operatively.

Unique from the previously discussed congenital lung lesions, thoracoscopic management is actually contraindicated for CLE as the overinflated lobe limits access to the chest. This makes thoracoscopic dissection in the neonate difficult and dangerous for patients with these lesions [22, 33, 34].

2.2 Malignancies

Malignancy of the pediatric chest is a rare event that when present should prompt consideration of pulmonary resection along with adjuvant therapy, the latter of which is beyond the scope of this text. Malignancies can be primary, most often pleuropulmonary blastoma, or more frequently metastatic. Metastatic disease most often results from osteosarcoma, Wilms tumor, and hepatoblastoma. Thoracoscopic intervention has been compared with open resection in this population, with thoracoscopic wedge resection now representing the most common therapeutic modality.

2.2.1 Pleuropulmonary blastoma

Pleuropulmonary blastomas (PPBs), though infrequently occurring (estimated incidence is 25–50 cases per year in the United States), are the most common primary pediatric pulmonary malignancy. They are associated with DICER1-related disorders, which have been described in detail elsewhere [35]. For the purposes of this text, it should be noted that this affiliation can result in concurrent primaries outside of the lungs and that all children with PPBs should undergo a thorough workup for additional malignancy, which includes genetic testing for a DICER1 mutation. Children with PPBs present with nonspecific findings that most frequently include respiratory distress, chest pain, and fever. It is uncommon to identify a PPB in the asymptomatic child.

PPBs progress through well-defined stages, which allows for them to be categorized into three unique types, where each corresponds to a different prognosis (**Table 1**). They are categorized based on the presence of cystic and solid components. There is some debate as to whether a type 1 lesion may regress (Type 1r) through the loss of malignant tissue. The controversy is that it is unclear whether these masses ever possessed a malignant component to begin with. Regardless, these lesions seem to be clinically insignificant, as the small number of patients who died after detection of a Type 1 mass experienced progression to Type 2 or 3 rather than Type 1r. No such regression has ever been described in Type 2 or 3 lesions (**Table 2**).

In comprehensive analyses of the PPB Registry, only type and metastases were identified as prognostic factors. Smaller cohort series have also suggested that the ability to achieve complete surgical resection may be prognostic, though this is debated. DICER1 mutations, found in up to two-thirds of patients, are common but definitively not prognostic. Nearly one-third of patients have a family member with a diagnosis within the DICER1 syndrome, including Wilms tumor, stromal tissue tumors, thyroid malignancy, cervical rhabdomyosarcoma, renal sarcoma, and pulmonary sequestration, to name a few [36].

A consensus on surgical management is not currently available, but reviews exist to guide the surgeon's approach and surveillance. Consideration should be given to the fact that these lesions may be mistaken for the previously described benign CPAMs, and that PPBs may progress from surgically amenable cystic masses (Type 1) to lethal metastatic disease with solid components (Type 2 or 3) if not managed promptly. The clinical feature best used for distinguishing CPAM from PPB is a systemic feeding vessel. But as has been stated previously, this not always found on imaging. Prenatal detection and pulmonary hyperinflation have also been suggested for their association with CPAM over PPB. On the other hand, multi-lobar or bilateral abnormalities,

	Type 1	**Type II**	**Type III**
Tissue type	Purely cystic	Cystic & solid	Purely solid
Frequency	1/3 of diagnoses	1/3 of diagnoses	1/3 of diagnoses
Age at diagnosis	Median: 8 months 95% by 36 months	Median: 35 months 95% by 81 months	Median: 41 months

Table 2.
Comparison of pleuropulmonary blastoma types.

complex cystic tissue, and mediastinal shift are all associated with PPB over CPAM. All children with cystic lung lesions should be considered for DICER1 testing to further assess their risk [37].

Patients with Type 1 disease are curatively managed with surgery alone when resection with negative margins and no tumor spillage is achieved. A wedge resection is most common, though lobectomy or other larger resections may be indicated for lesions with central, hilar, or multifocal involvement. Most authors have advocated for an open approach to the management of these lesions given the risk associated with tumor spillage. Smaller lesions, however, can be approached thoracoscopically by the surgeon adept in minimally invasive techniques [38].

Patients with Type 2 or 3 malignancy will often require adjuvant chemotherapy to minimize the resection necessary to achieve local control. Fortunately, PPBs are highly chemosensitive tumors, and neoadjuvant therapy can achieve a dramatic reduction in tumor size in patients for whom upfront surgery is deemed inappropriate. In general, the literature advocates for open resection in this population as increased size and tumor complexity make achieving a negative margin and spill-free resection difficult via a thoracoscopic approach. Lobectomy or pneumonectomy may be necessary to achieve adequate margins, and pleural surfaces should be taken *en bloc* with the implicated lung tissue.

In cases with extensive pleural spread, extra-pleural pneumonectomy may be necessary. This requires careful resection of the pleural surfaces, pericardium, diaphragm, and phrenic nerve along with division of the pulmonary hilar vessels. Children undergoing such extensive resection have a high rate of postoperative complications, most notably post-pneumonectomy syndrome. Unfortunately, PPB can progress or recur in patients with Type 2 or 3 disease, and both result in dramatically reduced survival [37].

The low incidence of childhood cancers is a defining challenge for the teams that manage them. A lack of robust clinical trials means that treatment algorithms are often driven by expert opinion and physician judgment based on retrospective and registry data. For PPB specifically, treatment options include surgery and chemotherapy as outlined here. The timing for each depends on the type and complexity of PPB. Ultimately, complete surgical resection is required for cure. Advancing the care and understanding of children with PPB will require cooperation across international study groups to organize prospective clinical trials.

2.2.2 Pulmonary metastatic disease

In addition to primary malignancy of the lung, pulmonary metastatic disease is an indication for surgical intervention of the infant or neonate. In fact, this is far *more* common than primary pulmonary malignancy. The most frequently implicated primaries are osteosarcoma, Wilms tumor, and hepatoblastoma (**Figure 5**). Metastasectomy has shown benefit for children with each of these malignancies, though pulmonary resection itself is not benign. The presence of uncontrolled primary disease and an inability to maintain adequate lung function after pulmonary resection are absolute contraindications to metastasectomy, regardless of primary.

Historically speaking, outcomes for children requiring pulmonary metastasectomy have been poor and difficult to study. Early literature was limited by its histologic heterogeneity, but more recent studies have illuminated some key points. We now know that staged bilateral resections are well tolerated and that the extent of metastasis is not an absolute contraindication to metastasectomy. This is largely the result

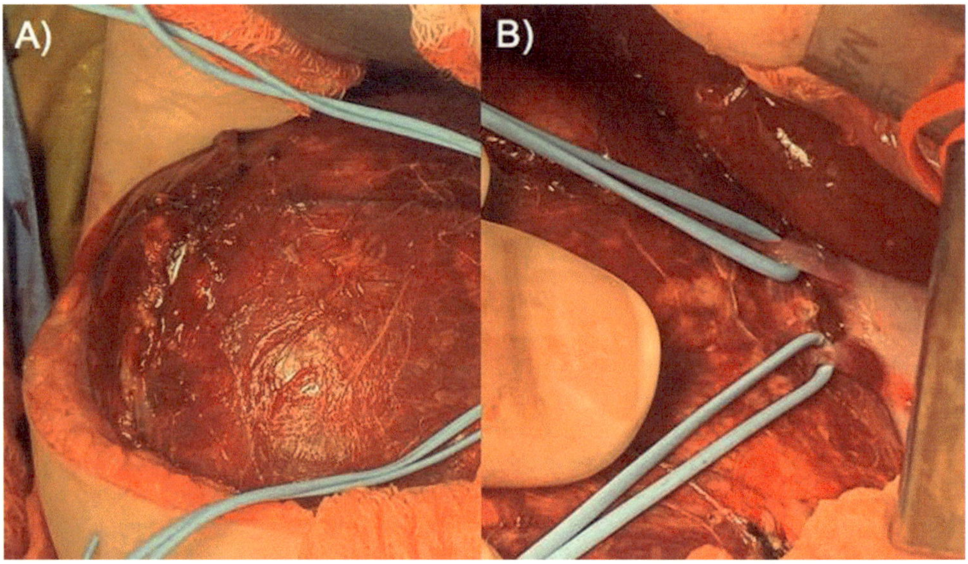

Figure 5.
A) Wilms tumor of the right kidney with B) blue vessel loops encircling the tumor's venous outflow.

of the now frequently utilized pulmonary wedge resection, which permits multiple lesions from both lungs to be excised while preserving non-diseased lung tissue. From a diagnostic perspective, CT has long been the gold standard for detecting pulmonary nodules. CT, however, lacks specificity and is unable to distinguish benign from malignant nodules. In the absence of tissue biopsy, this can lead to false positives and unnecessary surgical interventions [39]. Thus, thoracoscopy has a role in both therapy and diagnostic biopsy.

Wilms tumor is the most common pediatric solid tumor malignancy. Despite overall excellent outcomes for children with this diagnosis, patients with pulmonary metastasis fare poorly. Wilms tumor is responsive to radiotherapy, so whole lung radiation is commonly used for the management of pulmonary metastasis. In patients who do not respond to initial chest radiation, the Children's Oncology Group (COG) advocates diagnostic biopsy of lung nodules to minimize further exposure to toxic therapy in the cohort of patients with benign lesions. Minimally invasive approaches to metastasectomy are widely accepted in this cohort.

Hepatoblastoma also has dramatically decreased survival in children with pulmonary metastasis. Hepatoblastoma is sensitive to chemotherapy, and metastasectomy has been shown to be effective. Thus, the COG recommends a combined approach with neoadjuvant chemotherapy and subsequent total resection of the primary tumor and any pulmonary metastasis. Minimally invasive approaches to metastasectomy are widely accepted.

High-grade osteosarcoma accounts for roughly 5% of childhood malignancy. An important predicator of survival in this population is the presence of metastasis, and the lungs are the most common site for distant spread of malignancy. Though up to 10% of pulmonary metastasis are expected to regress with neoadjuvant chemotherapy, the remainder require surgical resection [40]. Interestingly, the timing of pulmonary metastasis is an important prognostic factor in children with osteosarcoma. Patients who experience pulmonary metastasis during chemotherapy have the worst survival [41].

Unlike metastasectomy for Wilms tumor or hepatoblastoma, there has historically been vigorous debate about the use of thoracoscopic resection in patients with osteosarcoma. The discussion has hinged on the fact that direct palpation of the lung via thoracotomy had been shown to detect osteosarcoma metastases that were not identified on CT. The impact of such lesions on survival, however, was not well understood and most treatment was based on surgeon judgment.

Recently, though, a multi-institutional collaborative group compared overall and disease-free survival in patients with metastatic osteosarcoma undergoing thoracoscopy and thoracotomy. They found equivalent overall and pulmonary disease-free survival in patients with oligometastatic pulmonary disease. Thoracoscopy, however, was associated with inferior overall survival when including patients with greater pulmonary burden. Ultimately, further investigation is still needed to determine the best strategy for treating osteosarcoma patients with pulmonary metastasis [42, 43]. Work in this area is ongoing, and the Children's Oncology Group has launched a randomized controlled trial comparing thoracoscopic interventions with bilateral staged thoracotomies in children and adolescents with oligometastatic osteosarcoma [44].

In conclusion, though children with solid tumors fare much better than in decades prior, pulmonary metastases still portend worse outcomes, regardless of primary histology. Surgery has a role to play in both diagnostic and therapeutic settings. Thoracoscopy is widely accepted for most metastasectomies, but evidence is limited on the potential benefits of lung palpation via thoracotomy in patients with osteosarcoma who may have radiographically undetectable pulmonary lesions.

2.3 Diagnostic dilemmas

In some groups of children, pulmonary resection is indicated due to diagnostic dilemmas. These typically occur when nodules or consolidations of unknown etiology develop and may represent malignancy or infection. This is observed in children requiring hematopoietic stem cell transplantation and immunosuppression. In these patients, such radiographic findings could result from infectious complications from their immunotherapy, progressive disease burden, or less frequently graft-versus-host disease. Thoracoscopic wedge resection with pathologic investigation of such ambiguous lesions is appropriate, as the potential for infection and malignancy have been described throughout this chapter [16, 19, 23, 25].

Another challenging situation occurs in the neonate suspected to have alveolar capillary dysplasia with misalignment of the pulmonary veins (ACD/MPV), which results from premature arrest of pulmonary development [45]. Although rare, the diagnosis should be considered in a neonate with unexplained persistent pulmonary hypertension (PPHN) [46]. Presentation is variable, but most infants have early onset respiratory distress [47]. Others will have a delayed presentation weeks to months after delivery [48]. A variety of coincidental defects in the cardiovascular, gastrointestinal, and urogenital systems have been documented [49]. Chest radiographs may demonstrate diffuse haziness or ground glass opacities but are frequently read as normal [50]. Echocardiograms can be useful for evaluation potential cardiac causes of PPHN.

Children with early onset symptoms typically demonstrate transient response to vasodilators, mechanical ventilation, and extra-corporeal membrane oxygenation but ultimately deteriorate and succumb to their disease without a transplantation [51–53]. Definitive diagnosis depends on surgical biopsy and tissue review by an experienced pediatric pathologist. Diagnostic clarity is essential in these cases as the prognosis is poor and early goals of care conversations are required.

3. Lobectomy considerations for infants and neonates

Thoracoscopic pulmonary resections are a well-described alternative to more invasive approaches to lung surgery in the adult and adolescent population. As has been described throughout this chapter, there is broad applicability of this approach to the infant and neonatal population with congenital or malignant abnormalities of the chest. Many of the same considerations from adult surgery apply, but a few are unique to the pediatric population. They are outlined here.

3.1 Lung isolation

Single lung ventilation is often necessary for successful thoracoscopic intervention as the lung is unable to be manually retracted. In adults and adolescents, there are a variety of options available to achieve this, including selective mainstem intubation, double lumen endotracheal tubes, Univent endotracheal tubes, and bronchial blockers. Neonates and infants, however, have smaller thoracic anatomy, which precludes the use of double lumen endotracheal or Univent tubes. Thus, selective mainstem intubation or bronchial blockers are required, though neither provides the same effectiveness as double lumen endotracheal tubes [54].

A major limitation to mainstem intubation is that the anesthesiologist cannot quickly change between single and two-lung ventilation as can be done with a double lumen device. Instead, they must reposition the endotracheal tube, which can result in accidental extubation. It should also be noted that mainstem intubation is particularly difficult on the left side, owing to the more acute angle of this bronchus.

Bronchial blockers can be used as an alternative to mainstem intubation. There are several candidate devices, including Fogarty catheters, pulmonary artery catheters, or the Arndt endobronchial blocker. Each of these can be used to occlude the bronchus on the operative side. The risk here is that the device becomes dislodged during the operation and occludes the tracheal lumen causing inadequate ventilation.

These considerations, although important, should not be prohibitive. Just as we advocate for neonatal thoracoscopic intervention in the hands of a skilled minimally invasive surgeon, so too attention should be placed on selecting an appropriately trained anesthesia staff with skills in neonatal intraoperative management. Such circumstances are a prerequisite for success during minimally invasive thoracic surgery of the infant or neonate [54].

3.2 Anatomic principles of lobectomy

In general, the anatomic principles of lobectomy are similar in neonates, adolescents, and adults. Only the necessary amount of lung for negative margins should be resected to maintain pulmonary function. Care should be taken to operate in an atraumatic fashion and to achieve hemostasis before closure. Respect for the anatomic boundaries and plains of the lungs is paramount. The neonatal circulation has a much smaller overall blood reserve, so volume losses can be detrimental. It is generally safer to take vessels at the segmental level instead of main trunks, and this is more easily done thoracoscopically.

In patients undergoing nonanatomic resections, either due to incorporation of multiple lobes into the lesion, or the presence of fissure fusion, the Ligasure has been recommended to complete a multi-segmentectomy [6].

3.3 Thoracoscopic techniques

Thoracoscopic lobectomy was first described in children by Steve Rothenberg for management of neonates with asymptomatic prenatally diagnosed lesions. He demonstrated that the skilled minimally invasive surgeon could safely and efficaciously apply thoracoscopic surgery to the small child in need of therapeutic lobectomy. Prior to this, the small size of young infants left surgeons unsure if their working space would be adequate for the large instrumentation required to complete a thoracoscopic resection.

His initial discussion of the thoracoscopic approach to neonatal lobectomy was limited to the previously discussed congenital lung malformations, but it now has broader applicability to the malignancies also mentioned in this chapter. Here we outline the modern technical details, which are built on his original approach [7].

Patients are placed in the lateral decubitus position and single lung ventilation is achieved via any of the approaches previously described for neonates. The surgeon and their assistant stand anterior to the patient while facing the surgical monitor. The first trocar is inserted, typically with an open technique, via the appropriate intercostal space based on the planed resection. As with other forms of minimally invasive surgery, the surgeon should attempt to "triangulate" their target for maximum maneuverability with the thoracoscopic instruments (**Figure 6**). If necessary, pneumothorax can be induced via insufflation with CO_2. Two to three additional ports are placed under video guidance based on appropriate surgical planning. These will be used for the dissection instruments and sealing device, typically a curved bipolar.

The relevant fissures and lobar vessels are dissected and sealed using the electrocautery. Endoclips should be considered if the patient has a pulmonary sequestration, as care must be taken to ligate the systemic feeding artery. The bronchus is sharply divided and closed intracorporeally using the surgeon's preferred approach. This may include suturing or stapling. The former requires adeptness with intracorporal suturing, though the latter necessitates a larger incision. After completing the lobectomy, the upper incision is lengthened, and the lobe is withdrawn. If the specimen contains malignancy, special attention is given to avoid spillage. A chest tube is left in place.

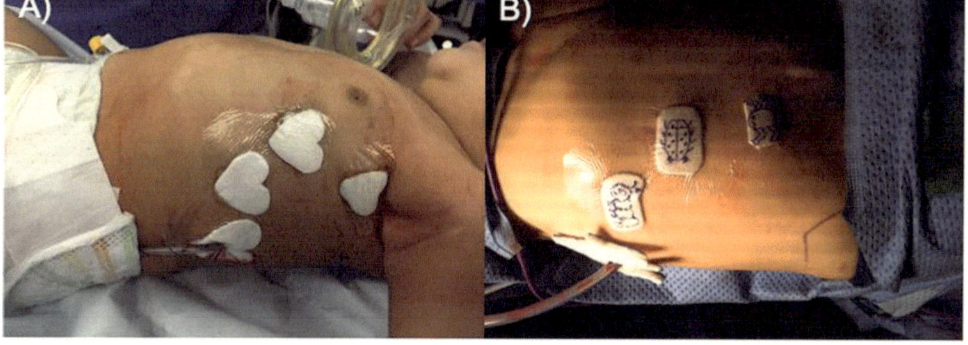

Figure 6.
A) Port placement for upper and B) lower lobectomy.

4. Pneumonectomy and other anatomic resections

4.1 Surgical principles

The principles of pneumonectomy, other anatomic resections, and wedge resections are similar in adults and children. Indications, as described above, include congenital pulmonary airway malformations, bronchopulmonary sequestrations, emphysema, and primary or metastatic malignancy. Lobectomy with en bloc tumor resection is the standard for patients with resectable cancers. Less extensive resections such as segmentectomy are chosen for patients who cannot tolerate lobectomy due to concern for limited pulmonary reserve [55].

The surgery is completed with the patient in the lateral decubitus position and the pleural space is entered through a posterolateral incision to provide exposure of the lung hilum. Inspection of the pleural space is performed; cytology and culture of any pleural fluid are completed as indicated. Arterial and venous supplies are identified, dissected, and divided at the hilum. Care should be taken not to injure the phrenic nerve when operating in the anterior hilum. Chest tubes are placed to drain residual fluid and support expansion of the residual lung.

4.2 Redo surgery

Redo thoracoscopic surgery is fraught with challenges and requires a special attention to relevant anatomy [56]. Adhesions and scar tissue contribute to a difficult operative field, just as in the adult population [57, 58]. There is precedent for approaching redo operations of the neonatal chest thoracoscopically, and we support such a strategy based on individual surgeon judgment. Still, preparations should be in place in the event that the case must be converted to open [59]. In rare circumstances, an intrapericardial approach to lobectomy or pneumonectomy can be considered in the extremely hostile reoperative chest [60, 61].

5. Perioperative complications of thoracoscopic surgery in neonates and infants

The feasibility and safety of thoracoscopic intervention have been rigorously reviewed in the adolescent population. It has been shown that the approach is not associated with increased risk compared with open surgery, while maintaining the previously described benefits of minimally invasive surgery. It is less thoroughly described in the infant and neonatal population, though we have discussed the common indications and emerging body of evidence, which supports its use in appropriate circumstances.

Reports of major complications from infant and neonatal thoracoscopy are limited but are summarized by a 2018 review published in the European Journal of Pediatric Surgery. Limited reporting of complications, small sample sizes, and study heterogeneity prevent the calculation of definitive complication rates in this population. Reported rates likely underestimate the true incidence due to reporting bias. Increased reporting of complications along with longitudinal patient series is encouraged to promote increased understanding of outcomes in this area and to guide decision-making when operative indications are equivocal [62].

5.1 Bleeding

Bleeding is one of most common complications in infants and neonates undergoing thoracoscopic surgery. This is of particular importance in the pediatric population given the limited total blood volume. Careful communication with anesthesia is essential to ensure that appropriate blood volume is available at the beginning of a case. There are also several instruments available for management of the bleeding vessel or tissue, including Heme-o-lok clips, pretied ligatures such as the ENDOLOOP, and stapling devices. Energy sources can also be used to achieve hemostasis, with LigaSure, HARMONIC, and Ultrasonic shears being common examples. Care should be given to not damage surrounding tissue when achieving hemostasis with the application of heat, as this can result in its own set of complications, which ironically enough can include additional bleeding. Intracorporeal suturing is also an option [7]. Whatever the approach, rapid control of bleeding is essential and proceeding with a large open thoracotomy is sometimes necessary.

5.2 Air leak

Persistent air leak is another commonly encountered complication of thoracoscopic surgery in neonates and infants. There are no evidence-based guidelines available for the management of this problem. Individual reports have demonstrated success with insertion of a secondary surgical chest tube, which has typically resulted in air leak resolution within a few days. In cases where the air leak has continued, reoperation with closure of a defect may be required. Chemical pleurodesis is well described in the adult population, but use of such toxic agents is discouraged in the pediatric population. There are limited reports of "autologous blood patching" wherein a bolus of the patient's own blood is injected into the pleural cavity through their chest tube [63]. Finally, there is a report of endobronchial occlusion of valves [64].

5.3 Conversion to open

Conversion is an outcome that must be considered in all approaches to minimally invasive surgery, including thoracoscopy. Bleeding, poor visualization, lesion size, pulmonary congestion, dissection difficulty, and the presence of unexpected lesions are all potential causes of conversion [62].

6. Conclusions

Thoracoscopic lobectomy is a strategy for surgical management of a wide range of pulmonary diseases in infants and children. These include congenital malformations, malignancies, and infections. There are similarities to resection in the adult population, but important differences exist too. The unique anatomic and physiologic principles of pediatric patients must be considered during surgical planning. The outcomes of these resections depend primarily on the underlying pathology.

Conflict of interest

The authors declare no conflict of interest.

Author details

Elisabeth T. Tracy[1*] and Steven W. Thornton[2]

1 Division of Pediatric Surgery, Duke University Department of Surgery, Durham, North Carolina, USA

2 Duke University Department of Surgery, Duke University School of Medicine, Durham, North Carolina, USA

*Address all correspondence to: elisabeth.tracy@duke.edu

References

[1] Hc J. Über die Möglichkeit die Zystoskopie bei Untersuchung seröser Höhlungen anzuwenden. Münchener Medizinische Wochenschrift. 1910;**57**:2090-2092

[2] Walker WS, Carnochan FM, Pugh GC. Thoracoscopic pulmonary lobectomy. Early operative experience and preliminary clinical results. The Journal of Thoracic and Cardiovascular Surgery. 1993;**106**(6):1111-1117

[3] McKenna RJ Jr, Houck W, Fuller CB. Video-assisted thoracic surgery lobectomy: experience with 1100 cases. The Annals of Thoracic Surgery. 2006;**81**(2):421-425 discussion 5-6

[4] Swanson SJ, Herndon JE 2nd, D'Amico TA, Demmy TL, McKenna RJ Jr, Green MR, et al. Video-assisted thoracic surgery lobectomy: Report of CALGB 39802-A prospective, multi-institution feasibility study. Journal of Clinical Oncology. 2007;**25**(31):4993-4997

[5] Onaitis MW, Petersen RP, Balderson SS, Toloza E, Burfeind WR, Harpole DH Jr, et al. Thoracoscopic lobectomy is a safe and versatile procedure: Experience with 500 consecutive patients. Annals of Surgery. 2006;**244**(3):420-425

[6] Rothenberg SS. First decade's experience with thoracoscopic lobectomy in infants and children. Journal of Pediatric Surgery. 2008;**43**(1):40-44 discussion 5

[7] Rothenberg SS, Middlesworth W, Kadennhe-Chiweshe A, Aspelund G, Kuenzler K, Cowles R, et al. Two decades of experience with thoracoscopic lobectomy in infants and children: Standardizing techniques for advanced thoracoscopic surgery. Journal of Laparoendoscopic & Advanced Surgical Techniques. Part A. 2015;**25**(5):423-428

[8] Ceppa DP, Kosinski AS, Berry MF, Tong BC, Harpole DH, Mitchell JD, et al. Thoracoscopic lobectomy has increasing benefit in patients with poor pulmonary function: A society of thoracic surgeons database analysis. Annals of Surgery. 2012;**256**(3):487-493

[9] Priest JR, Williams GM, Hill DA, Dehner LP, Jaffe A. Pulmonary cysts in early childhood and the risk of malignancy. Pediatric Pulmonology. 2009;**44**(1):14-30

[10] Sfakianaki AK, Copel JA. Congenital cystic lesions of the lung: Congenital cystic adenomatoid malformation and bronchopulmonary sequestration. Reviews in Obstetrics and Gynecology. 2012;**5**(2):85-93

[11] MacSweeney F, Papagiannopoulos K, Goldstraw P, Sheppard MN, Corrin B, Nicholson AG. An assessment of the expanded classification of congenital cystic adenomatoid malformations and their relationship to malignant transformation. The American Journal of Surgical Pathology. 2003;**27**(8):1139-1146

[12] Adzick NS, Harrison MR, Glick PL, Golbus MS, Anderson RL, Mahony BS, et al. Fetal cystic adenomatoid malformation: Prenatal diagnosis and natural history. Journal of Pediatric Surgery. 1985;**20**(5):483-488

[13] Kane SC, Ancona E, Reidy KL, Palma-Dias R. The utility of the congenital pulmonary airway malformation-volume ratio in

the assessment of fetal echogenic lung lesions: A systematic review. Fetal Diagnosis and Therapy. 2020;**47**(3):171-181

[14] Kantor N, Wayne C, Nasr A. Symptom development in originally asymptomatic CPAM diagnosed prenatally: A systematic review. Pediatric Surgery International. 2018;**34**(6):613-620

[15] Casagrande A, Pederiva F. Association between congenital lung malformations and lung tumors in children and adults: A systematic review. Journal of Thoracic Oncology. 2016;**11**(11):1837-1845

[16] Downard CD, Calkins CM, Williams RF, Renaud EJ, Jancelewicz T, Grabowski J, et al. Treatment of congenital pulmonary airway malformations: A systematic review from the APSA outcomes and evidence based practice committee. Pediatric Surgery International. 2017;**33**(9):939-953

[17] PAMG S. Congenital pulmonary airway malformation. National Library of Medicine. 2021

[18] Nasr A, Bass J. Thoracoscopic vs open resection of congenital lung lesions: A meta-analysis. Journal of Pediatric Surgery. 2012;**47**(5):857-861

[19] Adams S, Jobson M, Sangnawakij P, Heetun A, Thaventhiran A, Johal N, et al. Does thoracoscopy have advantages over open surgery for asymptomatic congenital lung malformations? An analysis of 1626 resections. Journal of Pediatric Surgery. 2017;**52**(2):247-251

[20] Lawal TA, Gosemann JH, Kuebler JF, Gluer S, Ure BM. Thoracoscopy versus thoracotomy improves midterm musculoskeletal status and cosmesis in infants and children. The Annals of Thoracic Surgery. 2009;**87**(1):224-228

[21] Dingemann C, Ure B, Dingemann J. Thoracoscopic procedures in pediatric surgery: What is the evidence? European Journal of Pediatric Surgery. 2014;**24**(1):14-19

[22] Vu LT, Farmer DL, Nobuhara KK, Miniati D, Lee H. Thoracoscopic versus open resection for congenital cystic adenomatoid malformations of the lung. Journal of Pediatric Surgery. 2008;**43**(1):35-39

[23] Adzick NS. Management of fetal lung lesions. Clinics in Perinatology. 2003;**30**(3):481-492

[24] Kapralik J, Wayne C, Chan E, Nasr A. Surgical versus conservative management of congenital pulmonary airway malformation in children: A systematic review and meta-analysis. Journal of Pediatric Surgery. 2016;**51**(3):508-512

[25] Stanton M, Njere I, Ade-Ajayi N, Patel S, Davenport M. Systematic review and meta-analysis of the postnatal management of congenital cystic lung lesions. Journal of Pediatric Surgery. 2009;**44**(5):1027-1033

[26] Gulack BC, Leraas HJ, Ezekian B, Kim J, Reed C, Adibe OO, et al. Outcomes following elective resection of congenital pulmonary airway malformations are equivalent after 3 months of age and a weight of 5 kg. Journal of Pediatric Surgery. 2017 Oct 9:S0022-3468(17)30639-5. DOI: 10.1016/j.jpedsurg.2017.10.017. Epub ahead of print. PMID: 29108843

[27] Yang L, Yang G. Extralobar pulmonary sequestration with a complication of torsion: A case report

and literature review. Medicine (Baltimore). 2020;**99**(29):e21104

[28] Kunisaki SM. Narrative review of congenital lung lesions. Translational Pediatrics. 2021;**10**(5):1418-1431

[29] Macardle CA, Ehrenberg-Buchner S, Smith EA, Dillman JR, Mychaliska GB, Treadwell MC, et al. Surveillance of fetal lung lesions using the congenital pulmonary airway malformation volume ratio: Natural history and outcomes. Prenatal Diagnosis. 2016;**36**(3):282-289

[30] Liu C, Pu Q, Ma L, Mei J, Xiao Z, Liao H, et al. Video-assisted thoracic surgery for pulmonary sequestration compared with posterolateral thoracotomy. The Journal of Thoracic and Cardiovascular Surgery. 2013;**146**(3):557-561

[31] Demir OF, Hangul M, Kose M. Congenital lobar emphysema: Diagnosis and treatment options. International Journal of Chronic Obstructive Pulmonary Disease. 2019;**14**:921-928

[32] Mendeloff EN. Sequestrations, congenital cystic adenomatoid malformations, and congenital lobar emphysema. Seminars in Thoracic and Cardiovascular Surgery. 2004;**16**(3):209-214

[33] Singh R, Davenport M. The argument for operative approach to asymptomatic lung lesions. Seminars in Pediatric Surgery. 2015;**24**(4):187-195

[34] Rahman N, Lakhoo K. Comparison between open and thoracoscopic resection of congenital lung lesions. Journal of Pediatric Surgery. 2009;**44**(2):333-336

[35] Caroleo AM, De Ioris MA, Boccuto L, Alessi I, Del Baldo G, Cacchione A, et al. DICER1 syndrome and cancer predisposition: From a rare pediatric tumor to lifetime risk. Frontiers in Oncology. 2020;**10**:614541

[36] PDQ Pediatric Treatment Editorial Board. Childhood Pleuropulmonary Blastoma Treatment (PDQ®): Health Professional Version. 2022 Jun 8. In: PDQ Cancer Information Summaries [Internet]. Bethesda (MD): National Cancer Institute (US); 2002. PMID: 31593396

[37] Knight S, Knight T, Khan A, Murphy AJ. Current Management of Pleuropulmonary Blastoma: A Surgical Perspective. Children (Basel). 2019 Jul 25;**6**(8):86. DOI: 10.3390/children6080086. PMID: 31349569; PMCID: PMC6721434

[38] Schultz KAP, Williams GM, Kamihara J, Stewart DR, Harris AK, Bauer AJ, et al. DICER1 and associated conditions: Identification of at-risk Individuals and recommended surveillance strategies. Clinical Cancer Research. 2018;**24**(10):2251-2261

[39] Croteau NJ, Heaton TE. Pulmonary Metastasectomy in Pediatric Solid Tumors. Children (Basel). 2019 Jan 8;**6**(1):6. DOI: 10.3390/children6010006. PMID: 30626161; PMCID: PMC6352020

[40] Basile P, Greengard E, Weigel B, Spector L. Prognostic factors for development of subsequent metastases in localized osteosarcoma: A systematic review and identification of literature gaps. Sarcoma. 2020;**2020**:7431549

[41] Ahmed G, Zamzam M, Kamel A, Ahmed S, Salama A, Zaki I, et al. Effect of timing of pulmonary metastasis occurrence on the outcome of metastasectomy in osteosarcoma patients. Journal of Pediatric Surgery. 2019;**54**(4):775-779

[42] Lautz TB, Farooqui Z, Jenkins T, Heaton TE, Doski JJ, Cooke-Barber J, et al. Thoracoscopy vs thoracotomy for the management of metastatic osteosarcoma: A pediatric surgical oncology research collaborative study. International Journal of Cancer. 2021;**148**(5):1164-1171

[43] Lautz TB, Krailo MD, Han R, Heaton TE, Dasgupta R, Doski J. Current surgical management of children with osteosarcoma and pulmonary metastatic disease: A survey of the American pediatric surgical association. Journal of Pediatric Surgery. 2021;**56**(2):282-285

[44] Children's Oncology Group NCIN. Thoracotomy Versus Thoracoscopic Management of Pulmonary Metastases in Patients With Osteosarcoma. 2022. Available online:https://clinicaltrials.gov/ct2/show/NCT05235165

[45] Fan LL, Deterding RR, Langston C. Pediatric interstitial lung disease revisited. Pediatric Pulmonology. 2004;**38**(5):369-378

[46] Cassidy J, Smith J, Goldman A, Haynes S, Smith E, Wright C, et al. The incidence and characteristics of neonatal irreversible lung dysplasia. The Journal of Pediatrics. 2002;**141**(3):426-428

[47] Janney CG, Askin FB, Kuhn C 3rd. Congenital alveolar capillary dysplasia-An unusual cause of respiratory distress in the newborn. American Journal of Clinical Pathology. 1981;**76**(5):722-727

[48] Ahmed S, Ackerman V, Faught P, Langston C. Profound hypoxemia and pulmonary hypertension in a 7-month-old infant: Late presentation of alveolar capillary dysplasia. Pediatric Critical Care Medicine. 2008;**9**(6):e43-e46

[49] Sen P, Thakur N, Stockton DW, Langston C, Bejjani BA. Expanding the phenotype of alveolar capillary dysplasia (ACD). The Journal of Pediatrics. 2004;**145**(5):646-651

[50] Bishop NB, Stankiewicz P, Steinhorn RH. Alveolar capillary dysplasia. American Journal of Respiratory and Critical Care Medicine. 2011;**184**(2):172-179

[51] Steinhorn RH, Cox PN, Fineman JR, Finer NN, Rosenberg EM, Silver MM, et al. Inhaled nitric oxide enhances oxygenation but not survival in infants with alveolar capillary dysplasia. The Journal of Pediatrics. 1997;**130**(3):417-422

[52] Kelly LK, Porta NF, Goodman DM, Carroll CL, Steinhorn RH. Inhaled prostacyclin for term infants with persistent pulmonary hypertension refractory to inhaled nitric oxide. The Journal of Pediatrics. 2002;**141**(6):830-832

[53] Parker TA, Ivy DD, Kinsella JP, Torielli F, Ruyle SZ, Thilo EH, et al. Combined therapy with inhaled nitric oxide and intravenous prostacyclin in an infant with alveolar-capillary dysplasia. American Journal of Respiratory and Critical Care Medicine. 1997;**155**(2):743-746

[54] Tobias JD. Anaesthesia for neonatal thoracic surgery. Best Practice & Research. Clinical Anaesthesiology. 2004;**18**(2):303-320

[55] Sabiston DC, Sellke FW, Del NPJ, Swanson SJ. Sabiston & Spencer surgery of the chest. Philadelphia: Saunders/Elsevier. 2010

[56] Fabian T, Van Backer JT, Ata A. Perioperative outcomes of thoracoscopic reoperations for clinical recurrence of pulmonary malignancy. Seminars in Thoracic and Cardiovascular Surgery. 2021;**33**(1):230-237

[57] Elkhouly A, Pompeo E. Nonintubated subxiphoid bilateral redo lung volume reduction surgery. The Annals of Thoracic Surgery. 2018;**106**(5):e277-e2e9

[58] Igai H, Kamiyoshihara M, Kawatani N, Shimizu K. Thoracoscopic right upper lobectomy after an initial anatomic pulmonary resection of the lower lobe. Multimedia Manual of Cardiothoracic Surgery. 2017 Nov 14;**2017**. DOI: 10.1510/mmcts.2017.014. PMID: 29300072

[59] Yim AP, Liu HP, Hazelrigg SR, Izzat MB, Fung AL, Boley TM, et al. Thoracoscopic operations on reoperated chests. The Annals of Thoracic Surgery. 1998;**65**(2):328-330

[60] Dell'Amore A, Pangoni A, Cannone G, Terzi S, Zuin A, Rea F. Video-assisted left lower lobectomy with intrapericardial pulmonary vein isolation. Multimedia Manual of Cardiothoracic Surgery. 2020 Sep 25;**2020**. DOI: 10.1510/mmcts.2020.051. PMID: 33263365

[61] Abu Akar F, Yang C, Lin L, Min SJ, Jiang L. Intra-pericardial double sleeve uniportal video-assisted thoracoscopic surgery left upper lobectomy. Journal of Visualized Surgery. 2017;**3**:51

[62] Zoeller C, Ure BM, Dingemann J. Perioperative complications of video-assisted thoracoscopic pulmonary procedures in neonates and infants. European Journal of Pediatric Surgery. 2018;**28**(2):163-170

[63] Lillegard JB, Kennedy RD, Ishitani MB, Zarroug AE, Feltis B. Autologous blood patch for persistent air leak in children. Journal of Pediatric Surgery. 2013;**48**(9):1862-1866

[64] Toth JW, Podany AB, Reed MF, Rocourt DV, Gilbert CR, Santos MC, et al. Endobronchial occlusion with one-way endobronchial valves: A novel technique for persistent air leaks in children. Journal of Pediatric Surgery. 2015;**50**(1):82-85

Section 3

Robotic-Assisted Thoracoscopic Surgery (RATS) Lobectomy

Chapter 4

Principles of Pulmonary Lobectomy

Raghav Chandra and Alberto de Hoyos

Abstract

Robotic-assisted thoracoscopic surgery (RATS), an evolution of minimally-invasive video-assisted thoracoscopic surgery (VATS), has recently emerged as the standard of care approach for pulmonary lobectomy for lung cancer. Despite increased upfront costs, RATS provides high-resolution, three-dimensional visualization of the operative field and enhanced instrument maneuverability with greater degrees of freedom. Several studies have demonstrated that RATS is non-inferior to VATS and may be associated with more complete mediastinal lymph node dissection and reduced risk of open conversion, length of stay, and intraoperative blood loss. In this chapter, we discuss the fundamental principles of robotic-assisted pulmonary lobectomy, indications and advantages of a robotic approach, and our operative technique.

Keywords: robotic-assisted thoracoscopic surgery, lobectomy, lung cancer

1. Introduction

Advances in *r*obotic-*a*ssisted surgery have revolutionized surgical practice in multiple specialties including *t*horacic *s*urgery (RATS). In the context of resection for lung cancer with curative intent, lobectomy remains the standard of care and most lobectomies worldwide are now performed through a minimally invasive approach, either through *v*ideo-*a*ssisted *t*horacoscopic *s*urgery (VATS) or RATS [1]. *R*obotic-*a*ssisted *l*obectomy (RAL) is an evolution of VATS lobectomy that is becoming increasingly common. Its most remarkable benefits include improved visualization with magnified, high definition, three-dimensional imaging coupled with upgraded instrument maneuverability. RAL has become the standard procedure in many centers and has surpassed VATS as the procedure of choice for lobectomy in the United States [2]. Here, we describe the principles of robotic pulmonary lobectomy for lung cancer.

2. Fundamentals of the da Vinci robotic system

The da Vinci Surgical System is currently the only robotic system approved by the United States Food and Drug Administration (FDA) for lung surgery (Intuitive Inc., Sunnyvale, CA). While originally designed for cardiothoracic surgery and utilized for deep pelvic operations in urology and gynecology, the da Vinci system has become rapidly integrated into multiple disciplines including general abdominal surgery,

IntechOpen

otorhinolaryngology, colorectal surgery, and cardiothoracic surgery [3]. In 2018, more than 1 million robotic cases using the da Vinci surgical system were performed worldwide [4].

The da Vinci robotic system consists of three primary components. First is a master surgical console controlled by the primary surgeon. This console transmits the surgeon's commands to the robotic instruments through hand controls and foot pedals and offers high-resolution three-dimensional visualization of the patient's anatomy. Second, the patient cart holds the instruments and the camera that are introduced into the patient through ports and are controlled by the surgeon at the master console. Third, the vision cart, is a network system which connects the console to the patient cart and facilitates seamless transmission of inputs from the surgeon at the console to the instruments on the patient, filtering out the natural tremor of the human hand [5]. A second optional console allows tandem surgery and training of residents and surgeons. In thoracic surgical procedures, the two most commonly utilized systems are the SI and the newer XI system. Compared with the older SI version, the XI system is more compact, and has thinner arms, longer instruments, and a swing beam that facilitates a greater range of motion and camera placement in any of the four ports for improved access to all areas of the chest [4].

While the advantages of VATS over traditional thoracotomy for pulmonary resection are well-documented (reduced postoperative pain, faster recovery, reduced risk of postoperative complications such as air leaks, pneumonia, or arrhythmias), comparisons between RATS and VATS are under active investigation [6]. Inherently, RATS allows for high-resolution 3D visualization of the structures in the thoracic cavity and enhanced range of motion and ergonomics compared with traditional straight and rigid thoracoscopic instruments. These advantages in turn allow for easier and complete mediastinal lymphadenectomy and precise vessel dissection [7, 8]. A recent clinical trial of 83 resectable NSCLC cases randomized to RATS vs. VATS demonstrated no difference in the rates of perioperative complications, operative time, or length of stay. However, the median number of sampled lymph node stations, and hilar and mediastinal nodal harvest were significantly greater in the RATS arm [9]. Additionally, a large meta-analysis of 18 studies with more than 11,000 patients demonstrated that RATS was non-inferior to VATS with respect to postoperative mortality, operative time, and overall or disease-free survival [10]. RATS was associated with significantly lower incidence of conversion to open, complication rate, chest tube duration, length of stay, reduced blood loss, and higher nodal harvest [10]. Conversely, RATS is associated with higher upfront investment and overall costs than VATS, which may preclude its widespread use at smaller institutions [10].

3. Indications for robotic pulmonary lobectomy and patient selection

The National Comprehensive Cancer Network (NCCN) and other society guidelines recommend surgical resection for Stage I and II diseases, and select cases of Stage III disease [11]. Lobectomy with hilar and mediastinal nodal sampling or dissection is the standard of care for oncologic resection, either RATS or VATS [12]. Patients should be evaluated preoperatively in standard fashion to define oncologic staging with an intravenous contrast enhanced computerized tomography (CT) scanning of the chest and abdomen, positron emission tomography (PET), and endobronchial ultrasound (EBUS) or mediastinoscopy, reserving brain magnetic resonance (MR) imaging for select cases [12]. Preoperative pulmonary function tests should be performed to ascertain adequate postoperative pulmonary reserve [13]. Indeed, a recent Society of Thoracic Surgeons database study demonstrated that RATS may be associated with decreased postoperative pulmonary complications in high-risk patients with limited pulmonary function, further highlighting the potential value of this approach [14].

3.1 Case selection

Robotic lobectomy is a challenging and high-stakes operation for novice robotic surgeons. It is recommended that surgeons begin their robotic experience with Level I operations (small mediastinal masses, wedge resection, and pleural and lymph node biopsies) before attempting more complex cases. Once some experience has been acquired, the surgeon should perform Level II operations (thymectomy for myasthenia gravis, diaphragm plication, mid-esophageal leiomyoma, chest wall resection) before proceeding to Level III operations (anatomic pulmonary resections, esophagectomy). When beginning to perform robotic assisted pulmonary resections, it is important for the surgeon and the surgical team to carefully select the cases to optimize the learning curve and patient outcomes. Cerfolio et al. suggested the following patient and tumor characteristics that make the initial pulmonary anatomic resections easier and safer [15].

- Tumor <5 cm
- No calcification of lymph nodes
- Peripherally located mass
- Normal bronchoscopy
- No other nodules in lung that need to be identified or resected
- CT scan suggestive of complete fissures
- Located in lower lobes
- No previous radiation
- No previous ipsilateral chest surgery

Once the surgeon and the team have acquired experience with "straightforward" cases, more challenging operations can be introduced, including sleeve lobectomy, segmentectomies, and pneumonectomies. Prior VATS experience with these operations facilitates skill acquisition and confidence, although not absolutely necessary.

4. Relevant anatomy

A deep knowledge of the pulmonary anatomy, and particularly, the spatial relationship between the hilar structures (arteries, veins, airways) and their potential variations, is needed to perform any lobectomy or segmentectomy safely. During a thoracotomy, the surgeon is positioned anteriorly or posteriorly and views the hilum from either the anterior or the posterior direction. In VATS and RAL, the camera approaches the hilum from a caudal direction and the surgeon needs to compensate mentally for this in order to safely conduct the operation. Avoiding misidentification of structures and attention to aberrant or variable anatomy are also of paramount importance to prevent injury that can force conversion to an open operation. In addition, an in-depth knowledge of the vascular anatomy and its variations is extremely helpful when performing technically difficult or challenging cases. Knowing the safe areas for vascular dissection can make a difficult case much simpler and safer.

5. Positioning and anesthesia

Upon arrival to the operating room (OR), patients undergo general endotracheal anesthesia with placement of a double-lumen endotracheal tube. This permits single-lung ventilation during the operation to optimize intraoperative view. The patient is placed in lateral decubitus position and a mild degree of flexion is introduced to the operating table to increase the space available between the ribs and to displace the hip from the chest taking care to maintain the chest in horizontal position. The patient is secured to the table, all pressure points are padded, and the arms are placed in neutral position to prevent stretch injury to the nerve and joints. Arterial line, bean bag, Foley catheter, and axillary rolls are not mandatory, and are used selectively. The patient's chest is prepped with antiseptic solution and sterilely draped. The surgeon's master console is typically near the patient's feet or head, and monitors are positioned in front and behind the patient. An assisting surgeon is positioned on one side of the patient for bedside assistance.

6. Operative technique

6.1 Analgesia and anesthetic technique

Patients scheduled for RAL are typically enrolled in an enhanced recovery pathway protocol. Preoperative analgesia medications include acetaminophen 1000 mg, celecoxib 400 mg, and gabapentin 900 mg or pregabalin 300 mg orally in the preoperative holding area. Patients additionally receive a paraspinal nerve block by the anesthesia service or intercostal nerve block with plain or liposomal bupivacaine intraoperatively. Other adjuncts include dexamethasone 10 mg intravenously, intercostal cryo-nerve analgesia, On-Q pump, and intravenous ketorolac 15–30 mg at the conclusion of the case. Postoperatively patients receive a combination of oral acetaminophen, nonsteroidal anti-inflammatory drugs (NSAIDs), and opioids, reserving intravenous opioids as rescue for severe pain.

6.2 Port placement

In general, five incisions are used for RAL, four robotic and one for the assistant. Non-stapling ports are 8 mm, and stapling and the assistant ports are 12 mm. The following is a description of the port placement for a robotic right upper lobectomy with the da Vinci XI system. All ports are marked with sterile ink before making an incision, although slight changes are often necessary once the intrathoracic anatomy is visualized. Ports are carefully and methodically planned to maximize maneuverability of robotic instruments, optimize access to the critical structures, and avoid internal or external collisions. The tip of the scapula is identified and marked to serve as reference, in case emergent conversion to open thoracotomy is required, avoiding using the ports as part of the incision as they are too low. The carefully planned port incisions are made, and the appropriate trocars are placed (preferably, all robotic ports are placed along the 7th (upper and middle lobe) or 8th intercostal space (lower lobe)). The first port to be inserted is the camera port (Arm 3 for right upper lobectomy). This port is usually placed at the posterior axillary line one or two intercostal spaces inferior and anterior to the tip of the scapula. The thoracic cavity is inspected, and the remaining ports are placed under direct visualization. Arm 1 is placed 3 cm from the spine and one or two intercostal spaces below the tip of the superior segment of the lower lobe to allow unimpeded retraction and manipulation of the lung. This arm, in essence, functions as the exposure or retraction arm. Arm 2 is placed between Arms 1 and 3 or one intercostal space below. Arm 4 is placed as anteriorly as possible and just above the diaphragm. The assistant port is placed between Arms 3 and 4 in an isosceles triangular configuration to allow adequate working space for the bedside assistant. Warmed and humidified carbon dioxide is insufflated to a pressure of 5–8 mmHg through the access port to drive the diaphragm inferiorly and help with lung atelectasis. The robot can approach the operating room table perpendicular to the patient, after which the beam is rotated to the proper position. We utilize a zero-degree camera instead of a 30-degree camera due to its decreased torque, which reduces the chances of intercostal nerve injury [16].

6.3 Instrument selection

Most robotic lobectomies can be completed with three instruments and a stapler (**Figure 1**). For right-sided lobectomies, we utilize a tip-up fenestrated instrument in Arm 1 that serves as the lung retractor. In Arm 2, we utilize Cadiere forceps to manipulate the lung or tissue or a stapler to divide structures. In Arm 3, we place the camera. In Arm 4, we use a Maryland bipolar or curved bipolar dissector. Vascular

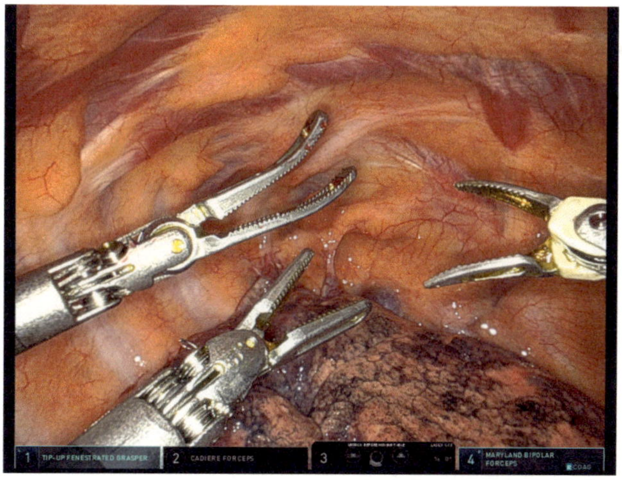

Figure 1.
Robotic lobectomy usually requires only three instruments and a stapler. From left to right the instruments are: Fenestrated tip-up, Cadiere forceps, and Maryland bipolar.

structures are divided with white loads, lung parenchyma with blue or green loads, and the bronchus with green or black loads. Black loads are reserved for thick tissues. Lower profile vascular staplers that are capable to fit through the 8-mm cannulas have received FDA approval and are scheduled to be released in the fall of 2022. All instruments are introduced slowly and under direct vision and positioned toward the apex of the chest to prevent injury to intrathoracic structures. Once in view, the surgeon at the master console can gain control of the instruments and commence the operation.

6.4 Initial assessment

The procedure begins by performing a thorough examination of the thoracic cavity including the chest wall, mediastinum, diaphragm, and the lung to determine if any unexpected abnormalities exist. The target lobe to be removed is visualized and the tumor identified, if possible. If no preoperative diagnosis is available, a wedge resection of the nodule is performed and submitted for frozen section analysis. While waiting for the results of the biopsy (usually 20–30 minutes), the next step of the procedure can be performed.

6.5 Mediastinal and hilar lymphadenectomy

A complete hilar and mediastinal nodal sampling or dissection can be performed in 15 minutes or less. Complete lymphadenectomy is of paramount importance for both adequate pathologic staging and to help expose the vascular structures of the hilum and facilitate their dissection and division. For accurate nodal count and pathologic staging, it is recommended that nodal tissue from one specific lymph node be submitted in one cup, either whole or in fragments as to not count fragments as individual lymph nodes. One cup represents one individual lymph node. Multiple nodes from one station are labeled sequentially (i.e., 7a, 7b).

6.5.1 Right side (9,8,7,10,11,4,2)

The inferior pulmonary ligament is divided from the diaphragm to the inferior pulmonary vein. For this step, robotic Arm 1 (fenestrated tip-up) is used to retract the lower lobe cephalad toward the superior chest and anteriorly. For optimal dissection and less bleeding, it is best to grasp the tissue around the lymph nodes with the Cadiere forceps and use the bipolar energy to cauterize the small feeding vessels around the node. If the node needs to be manipulated, it is best to incorporate the whole node to prevent fracturing and bleeding. Lymph nodes at stations 8 and 9 are removed. Arm 1 is then repositioned and retracts the lung medially and anteriorly to dissect the area of the mediastinum posterior to the pericardium, exposing additional level 8 nodes and the subcarinal space. The nodal tissue in station 7 can be removed incorporating several lymph nodes in the specimen, clearly exposing the left main bronchus and the esophagus. In this area, bronchial artery branches can cause troublesome bleeding and efforts should be placed in identifying and controlling these small vessels with electrocautery. Rolled sponges with a radiopaque marker should be available at all times to help keep the visual field clear of blood. The dissection continues cephalad toward the azygous vein, identifying and removing visible level 10 hilar lymph nodes usually located behind the airway. At this time, it is also recommended to identify the crotch between the right upper lobe (RUL) bronchus and the right lower lobe (RLL) bronchus. At this location, the interlobar node or the sump node or level 11 (superior interlobar node of Rouviere or sump node of Borrie) is dissected and removed, exposing the lower edge of RUL bronchus and the recurrent branch of the pulmonary artery (**Figures 2** and **3**). Arm 1 is then utilized to retract the RUL caudally to expose the superior hilum. This maneuver exposes stations 4 and 2 that lie in the triangle formed by the superior vena cava anteriorly, the trachea posteriorly and the azygos vein caudally (**Figure 4**). Rather than identifying individual nodes in this area, the entire lymph node packet at this location is dissected and removed and nodes can be separated at the back table (**Figure 5**). Care must be taken to identify and protect the vagus nerve at this location running along the trachea toward the tracheoesophageal groove. While looking at the superior hilum, additional level 10 nodes can be identified and removed adjacent to the azygos vein (**Figures 6** and **7**). Areas of dissection are checked for bleeding and gently pack with hemostatic agents.

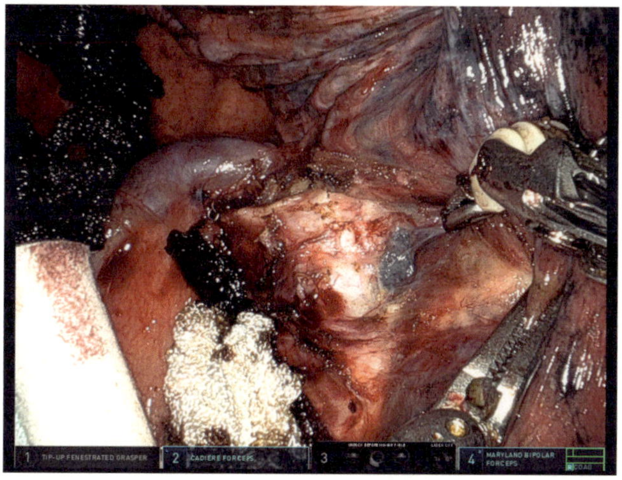

Figure 2.
The right upper lobe and bronchus intermedius are shown with the level 11 interlobar or sump node at the crotch.

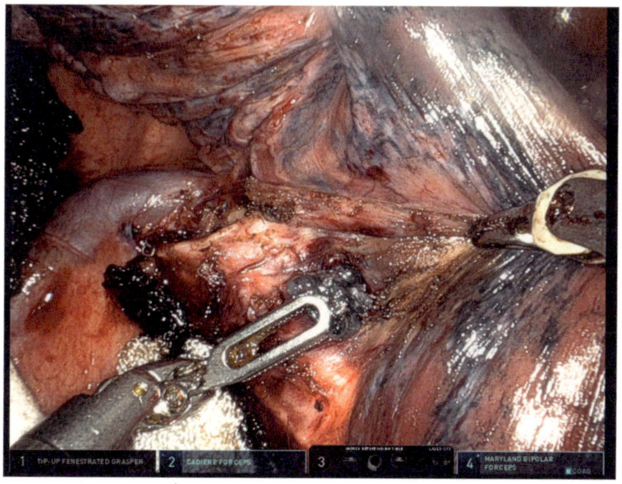

Figure 3.
Dissection of the interlobar or sump node exposes the recurrent branch of the pulmonary artery and is essential to get around the right upper lobe bronchus.

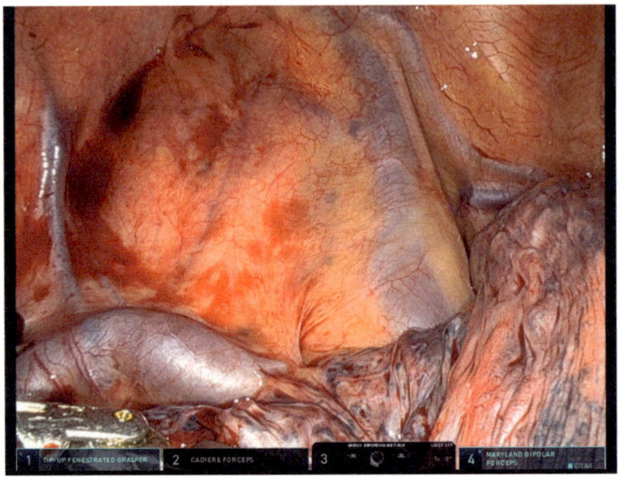

Figure 4.
Caudal retraction of the right upper lobe allows access to level 4 and 2 mediastinal nodes, located in the triangle formed by the superior vena cava (SVC) anteriorly, the trachea posteriorly, and the azygos vein caudally. The phrenic nerve is shown running along the SVC.

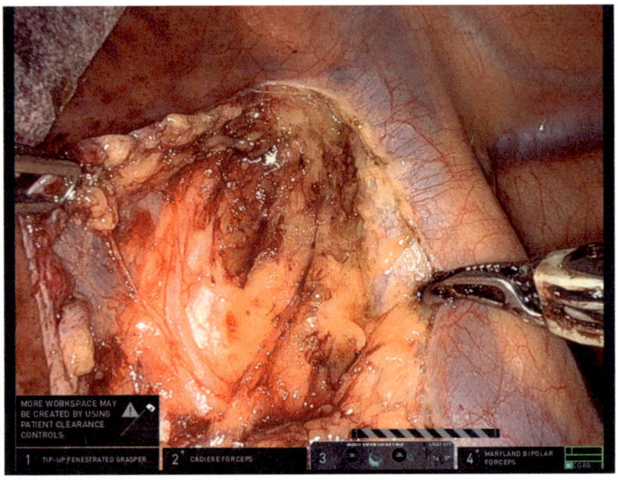

Figure 5.
The entire fat pad in this location is dissected removing several levels 4 and 2 lymph nodes together. These nodes can be separated and placed in individual cups on the back table.

6.5.2 Left side (9,8,7,10,5,6,11)

Similar steps are followed when performing lymphadenectomy for left-sided lung tumors. In this case, Arm 4 will be the lung retractor, while Arms 1 and 3 will be the dissecting instruments. The inferior pulmonary ligament is divided to identify and remove the lymph node on station 9. The node(s) in station 8 are dissected and removed. Subcarinal node dissection on the left side is more challenging than that on the right side and is facilitated, in a lower lobectomy, by division of the bronchus. Lymph nodes at station 7 are accessed in the space between the inferior pulmonary

DOI: http://dx.doi.org/10.5772/intechopen.107342

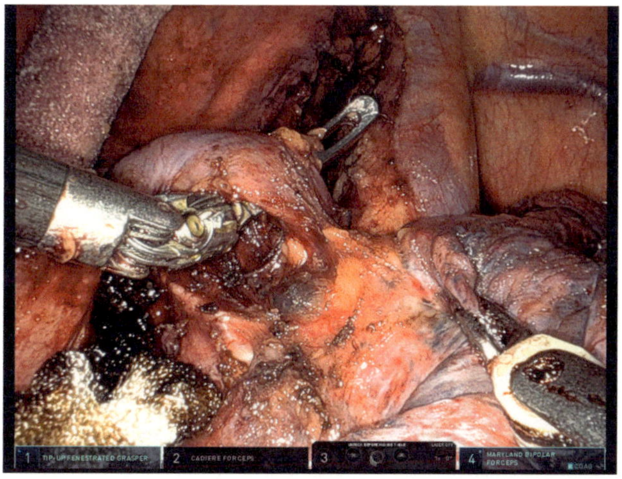

Figure 6.
Additional level 10 or hilar nodes can be dissected between the bronchus and the azygos vein. Elevating the azygos vein ensures all nodes in this area are removed.

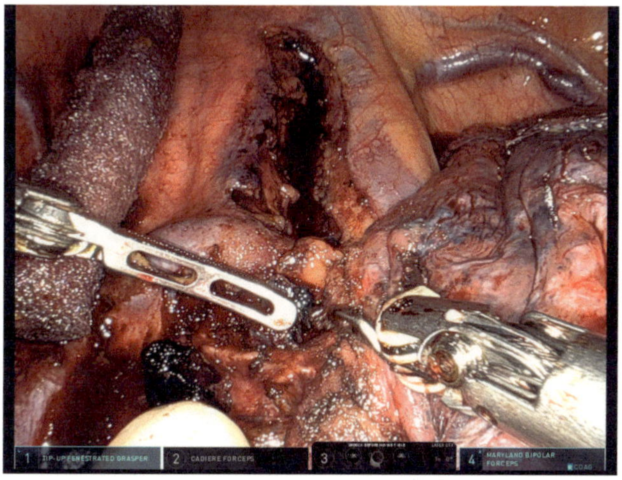

Figure 7.
Additional level 10 or hilar nodes dissected between right main bronchus and azygos vein.

vein and lower lobe bronchus, lateral to the esophagus and in front of the aorta. The lower lobe is retracted medially/anteriorly with Arm 4 during this process. Posterior level 10 and 11 lymph nodes can be dissected and removed at this time and are usually located next to the pulmonary artery at the cephalad end of the interlobar fissure. Finally, robotic Arm 4 is used to wrap around the left upper lobe and pressed it caudally and inferiorly to allow exposure of the superior hilum and dissection of stations 5 and 6. Care should be taken while working in the aortopulmonary window to avoid injury to the left recurrent laryngeal nerve. Station 2 L and 4 L cannot typically be accessed during left-sided lobectomies owing to the presence of the aortic arch, although on occasion 4 L nodes can be identified.

7. Right upper lobectomy

Once the mediastinal and hilar lymphadenectomy is completed, the operation can be performed in one of three ways: 1) traditional VATS approach from anterior to posterior, 2) in reverse order posterior to anterior beginning with the bronchus (bronchus first technique), or 3) superior hilar approach with division of the pulmonary artery (PA) vessels first. A certain degree of adaptability is necessary for performance of RAL as structures may be isolated and divided in a systematic orderly fashion or in the order that the patient's individual anatomy permits. Our preference is to minimize manipulating and flipping the lung as much as possible and therefore, we prefer the latter two options since the dissection started at the back of the lung for the lymphadenectomy.

Retraction of the right upper lobe caudally and inferiorly with Arm 1 helps to expose the superior hilum, which is the last step of the lymphadenectomy on the right side. The mediastinal pleura above the lung at this location is incised to expose the pulmonary vein branches anteriorly and the pulmonary artery branches posteriorly (truncus anterior and posterior branch). The 10R lymph node between the truncus branch and the superior pulmonary vein if visible should be removed or swept up toward the lung, which exposes the truncus branch. The truncus branch is dissected taking care to enter the vascular sheath or plane of Leriche, which makes the vessel dissection simpler and safer (**Figure 8**). At times the entire arterial blood flow to the RUL arises from a single trunk that can be divided with a single vascular load, but more commonly, the truncus anterior is separate from the posterior and the recurrent branch. The truncus is dissected circumferentially with a Cadiere forceps (Arm 4) placing a vessel loop around the artery (**Figure 9**). Temptation must be resisted to use the Maryland or curve bipolar dissector to perform this step as a catastrophic injury to the back wall of the artery may result due to their pointed tip. A tip-up stapler with a vascular load is introduced through arm 2 or 4 and the vessel divided (**Figure 10**). We prefer to avoid placing the stapler from a posterior approach as currently it requires a 12-mm cannula and is more likely to cause persistent pain due to the narrower rib spaces. The posterior

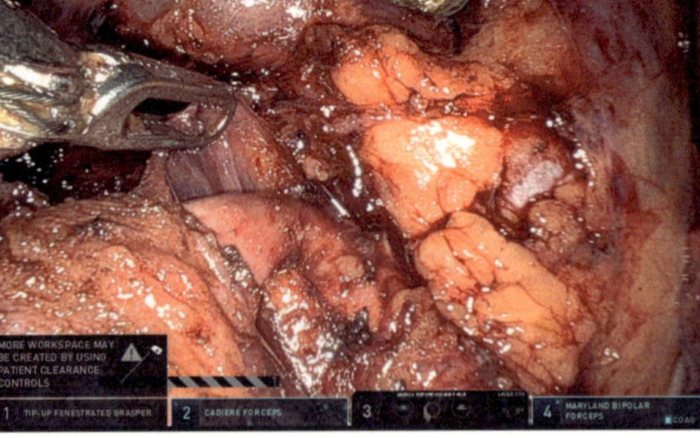

Figure 8.
The arterial truncus to the right upper lobe is shown. The perivascular sheath is incised to enter the plane or space of Leriche. Dissection in this plane makes isolation and division of the vessels easier and safer.

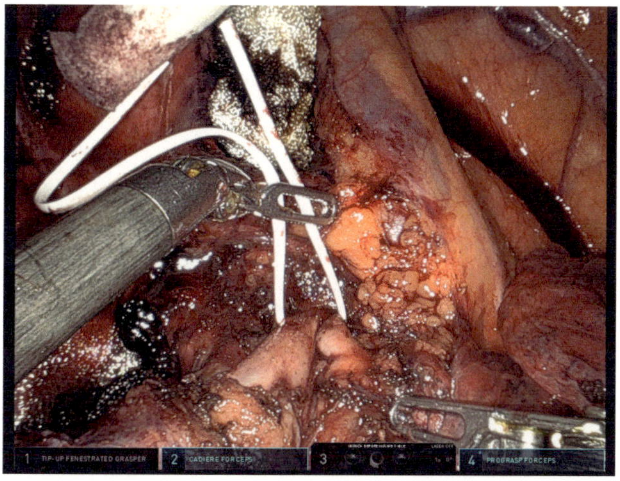

Figure 9.
The arterial truncus has been dissected circumferentially, and the vessel is elevated with a vessel loop at the common origin of the branches.

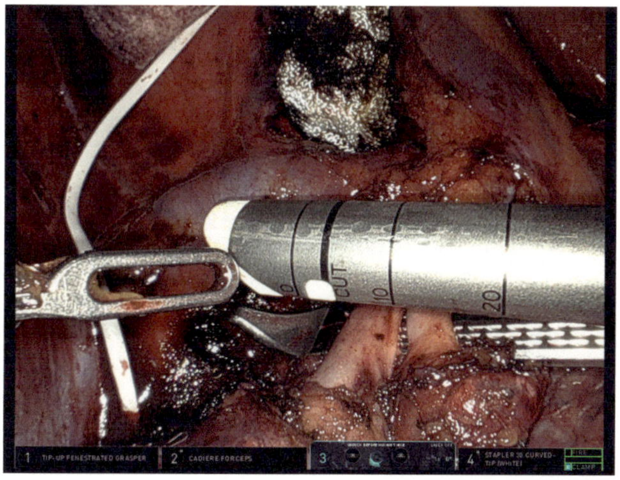

Figure 10.
Stapling of the arterial truncus. The anvil with a ski tip is placed under the artery taking care to avoid lifting or stretching the artery to avoid injury.

branch to the RUL, if present between the RUL bronchus and the truncus anterior, is similarly dissected and divided, further exposing the RUL bronchus. Often there is a level 10 or level 11 lymph node at this location and its removal makes vascular isolation and division simpler and safer. The RUL is returned to its anatomic position and with Arm 1 is displaced superiorly, medially, and anteriorly to expose the RUL bronchus and the bronchus intermedius. Since the sump node at this location has already been removed during the lymphadenectomy, the recurrent branch of the pulmonary artery is easily recognized if present. At times, two recurrent branches are present or origin from a6 must be recognized in order to avoid injury. A branch of the pulmonary vein can also be identified at this location. A complete major fissure or division of the posterior aspect of the fissure can help with the exposure and dissection and division

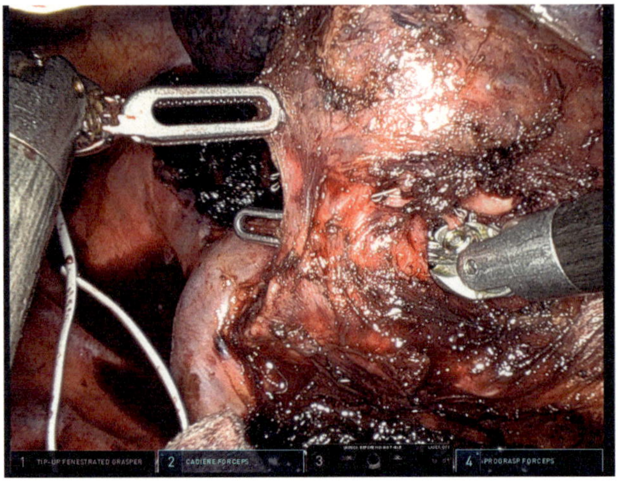

Figure 11.
The right upper lobe bronchus is dissected by placing a Cadiere forceps in front of the bronchus. Since the arterial truncus has already been divided, there is little risk of vascular injury during this maneuver. In the bronchus first technique, this step requires meticulous technique passing the instrument in front of the bronchus to avoid injury to the vessel.

of these vascular structures. Additional level 11 lymph node removal around the origin of the vessels can facilitate vascular dissection and division. Since the pulmonary artery branches in the upper hilum have already been divided, the RUL bronchus can safely be encircled with a vessel loop by passing the Cadiere forceps from the anterior port or Arm 4 (**Figure 11**). A stapler with a green load is exchanged for the Cardiere forceps, and the RUL bronchus is divided (**Figure 12**). At times, the recurrent branch of the pulmonary artery is easier to divide once the bronchus has been transected (13). Division of the RUL bronchus allows to elevate the RUL and expose the posterior aspect of the minor fissure and the pulmonary artery to the right middle lobe (RML) and right lower lobe (RLL) (**Figure 13**). Dissection on the plane of the artery helps

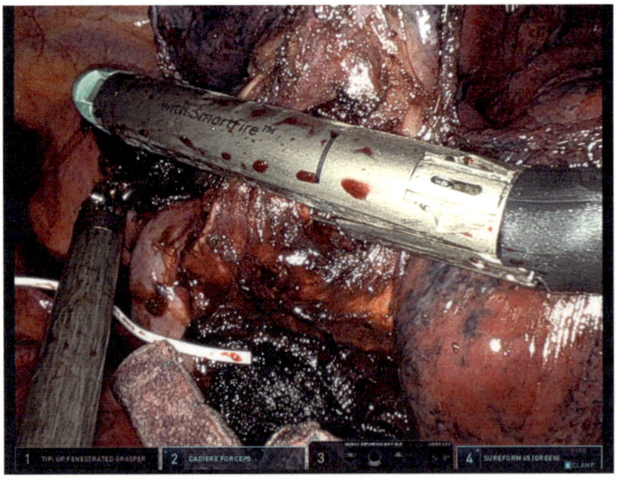

Figure 12.
Bronchi are usually divided with green loads unless they are thick due to prior chemotherapy or radiation. In this situation, a black load may be necessary.

DOI: http://dx.doi.org/10.5772/intechopen.107342

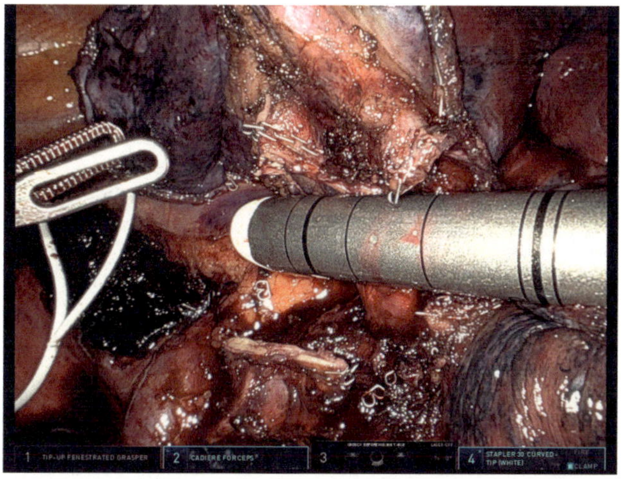

Figure 13.
Division of the right upper lobe bronchus can expose a second recurrent branch of the pulmonary artery to the upper lobe as in this case.

identify the origin of the RML branch of the pulmonary artery and safe division of the posterior aspect of the minor fissure with a stapler introduced through port 2. During completion of the minor fissure, the RUL should be lifted up to ensure that the divided RUL bronchus is included in the specimen (**Figure 14**). Additional blue loads are fired along the minor fissure until the RUL vein is encountered. Once the vein is reached, the branches to the RUL are encircled and divided with a vascular load, leaving the RML in place. Alternatively, if vein visualization is not clear, the lung can be retracted posteriorly with arm 1 and the superior pulmonary vein exposed. The bifurcation between the RUL and RML veins is developed by dissecting it off the underlying pulmonary artery (**Figure 15**). The branches to the RUL are encircled with the vessel loop and divided

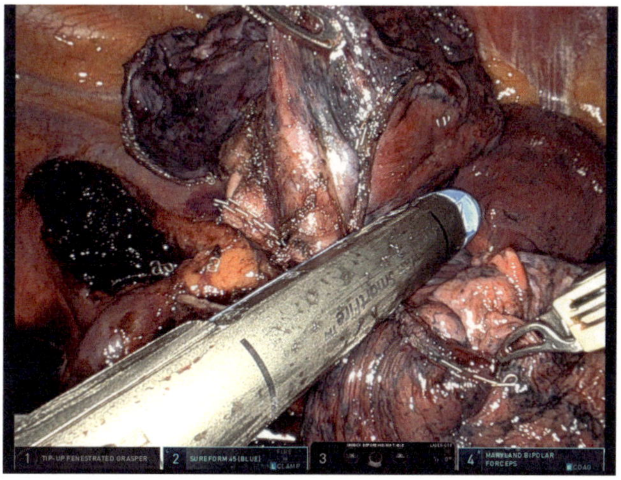

Figure 14.
Stapling of the minor fissure from posterior to anterior placing the stapler above the descending trunk of the pulmonary artery and its middle lobe branch. Care must be taken to avoid injury to the middle lobe vein.

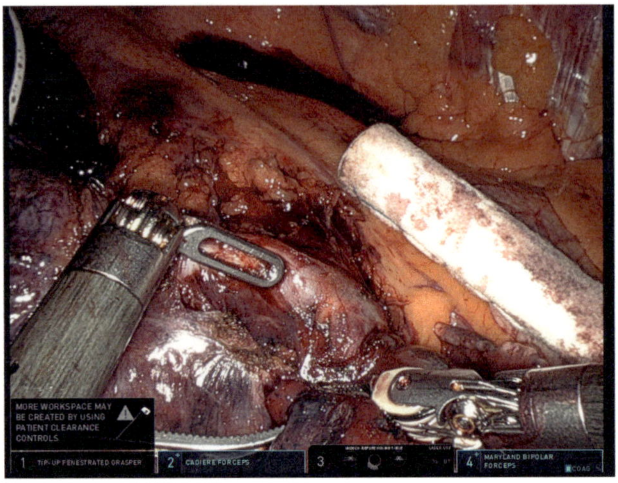

Figure 15.
View of the superior pulmonary vein showing the angle between the upper and middle lobe veins. Dissection posterior to the upper lobe branches is performed taking care to avoid injury to the pulmonary artery located posteriorly.

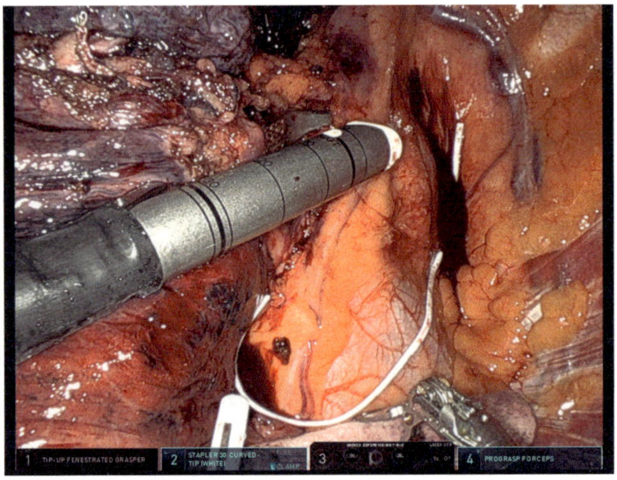

Figure 16.
Stapling of the superior pulmonary vein to the right upper lobe completing the lobectomy.

with a vascular load introduced through Arms 2 or 4 (**Figure 16**). The reminder of the minor fissure is divided completing the lobectomy.

On occasion, particularly after induction therapy or in the presence of adenopathy stuck to the truncus anterior, when arterial dissection is difficult, it is better to divide the upper lobe bronchus with scissors to get to a fresh plane on the artery rather than risk arterial injury. Once the dissection is completed, the bronchus is closed with interrupted sutures. Buttressing of the bronchial closure is encouraged after induction treatment.

The specimen is placed in a bag and extracted from the chest cavity through either the access port or the anterior port (Arm 4). The chest cavity is copiously irrigated with saline, hemostasis is ensured, and a single 24 Fr chest tube advanced into the pleural space. If more than usual oozing or bleeding is anticipated, a larger bore tube or a Blake drain is placed. The fascia and skin over the incision sites is closed in standard fashion.

8. Dealing with an incomplete fissure

In situations where the fissures are incomplete and thick, it is preferable to avoid dissecting it because this will result in bleeding from the lung parenchyma and prolonged air leaks. A better option in these situations is to perform a fissureless or tunnel technique approach to lobectomy [17, 18]. For all three fissures, the tunnel technique starts with dissection between the lobar veins and proceeds cephalad (bottom-to-top technique). This technique can be applied easier to lower and middle lobectomies as the dissection starts caudally by dividing the fissure between the lingula and the lower lobe in the left, or between the lower lobe and middle lobe in the right where there are no vascular structures to divide or at risk, but can also be performed for right upper lobectomy. The division of the caudal and anterior portion of the major fissure is taken to the pericardium between the superior and inferior pulmonary veins. At this point, the lung is retracted cephalad splaying open the divided portion of the fissure to expose the two veins and all the fat and lymph nodes are removed to expose the bronchus and the PA. If a lower lobectomy is being performed, the corresponding vein can be divided at this point, but it is not absolutely necessary. Next, dissection is continued between the bronchi (except for the horizontal fissure) and between the artery and the parenchyma. The lower lobe bronchus usually comes into view first. Dissection continues until a branch of the pulmonary artery to a basilar segment is identified. At this point, the basilar trunk of the pulmonary artery is identified and a plane of dissection or tunnel is established between the artery and the lung parenchyma above. Using Cadiere forceps, the tunnel is created between the anterior surface of the artery and the thick fissure. The ideal dissection plane is close to the artery gently dividing the flimsy connective tissue until the artery is free. Once this tunnel is 3–4 cm in length, the thick fissure is divided with a stapler introducing the anvil in the tunnel. Firing the stapler will open part of the incomplete fissure, and tunneling continues along the artery. The process is repeated until the top of the fissure is reached. Freeing the "exit" of the tunnel first makes the procedure much easier and safer as the anvil can be advanced beyond the exit point without any resistance or obstruction. On the left side the exit point is located at the artery, more specific, between the artery of the posterior segment (a2) of the upper lobe and the apex artery of the lower lobe (a6). The exit point is dissected by first dividing the fused top end of the fissure with a stapler and dissecting the artery at the superior hilum. On the right, the exit can be found at the secondary carina between upper lobe bronchus and bronchus intermedius. We have utilized this approach in a large number of patients without conversion for bleeding (manuscript in preparation). Once the entire fissure has been divided, access to any arterial branches becomes much safer and the operation can continue in seamless fashion.

9. Handling intraoperative bleeding during RAL

One of the most feared events in minimally invasive lobectomy is injury to the pulmonary artery. Cerfolio et al. reported an incidence of major vascular injury of

2.6% during RAL [19]. Novellis et al. reported an overall conversion rate of 6.2% for major robotic lung resections, of which 1.1% (4/338) were due to bleeding [20].

The most common and serious intraoperative bleeding complication during RAL is an injury to the PA. Most commonly these injuries occur during dissection of the artery and are easy to recognize as they occur directly at the point of dissection [21]. Injury can also occur at the time of blind dissection behind the artery or passage of the stapler [22]. In these instances, the pulmonary artery injury (PAI) is usually at the branch point resulting in a more proximal injury, which is more difficult to repair robotically. Most commonly, a central injury to the PA during RAL occurs during left upper lobectomy and is associated with dissection, isolation, and division of the truncus anterior, which is typically large in diameter and short in length.

The risk factors for PAI with robotic lung resection are similar to open or VATS procedures. The risk of PAI is increased in patients who have received induction chemo- and/or radiation therapy, larger tumors, and in the presence of calcified lymph nodes attached to the artery [23, 24]. Pulmonary vein injury is much less common than PAI and is more easily repaired using minimally invasive techniques and will not be discussed further.

The location of the PAI is the key to its management and deciding if it is possible to control the bleeding robotically or conversion to thoracotomy is required. In other words, can the bleeding be controlled and can the proximal PA be clamped safely? In our experience, repairing a PAI robotically is complex and is only feasible for surgeons with extensive experience in RATS and ideally in expert and high-volume centers that also have highly-trained surgical teams. There are essentially two PAI scenarios during RAL: First, the injury is located on the main PA or its proximal branches during upper lobectomy, or second, the injury is located on the lower or middle lobe arteries or on the distal branches of any lobe. The first step in both situations is to immediately control the bleeding with a sponge roll and pressure using the lung itself if possible, and resisting the urge to clamp the vessel with the robotic instruments [25].

Cerfolio et al. described the 4 *"P"'s* as the technique for the control of major vascular injury during RAL: *P*oise, *P*ressure, *P*reparedness, and *P*roximal control [19]. Preparedness can be further expanded to *P*revention of the injury and *P*reparedness of the team to respond to the catastrophic event [26]. A *sixth P* can be added as the vessel is usually repaired with *P*olypropilene suture.

9.1 The 5 "P"'S

Prevention First and foremost is Prevention. Prevention of major vascular injury requires complete and methodical dissection of the perivascular structures, avoiding undue traction of the vessel and being aware of branch points. The strategy of RAL usually starts with a wide mediastinal and hilar nodal dissection with the identification of the proximal or lobar vascular structures. This is followed by dissection of the smaller or segmental vascular branches once the perivascular N1 nodes have been removed and the spaces have been created for the safe passage of the instruments and the stapler. The use of vessel loops for elevation of the vessel and the use of tip-up staplers or guide catheters further decreases the chance of vascular injury. As a general rule, the branch of the pulmonary artery and the proximal portion of the artery giving rise to the branch should be completely dissected before any attempt is made to encircle the branch. This is facilitated by removing all N1 nodes at this location. Decreasing tension on the branch point during dissection and passage of instruments is an excellent technique for avoiding injury to the artery. In general, greater dissection of N1 nodes and perivascular structures leads to safer exposure and control of the pulmonary artery branches and prevention of catastrophic bleeding. The *"P"* for prevention is the most important of the 5 "P"'s.

Preparedness The surgical and the anesthesia teams need to prepare by performing drills such that each team member is assign a role and is ready in the event of vascular injury. It is the responsibility of the primary surgeon to organize and direct these drills for optimal outcomes in case of severe or catastrophic vascular injury. This requires dedicated anesthesia and nursing teams. Thoracotomy trays with several hand-picked vascular clamps must be in the room, and possibly opened and counted depending on the experience of the surgeon. Suture material (Prolene 4-0 and 5-0), pledgets and blood need to be also available.

Poise: Poise is the most critical response to a catastrophic vascular injury. The primary surgeon must remain as relaxed as possible in order to create a calm attitude and transmit confidence to all members of the surgical, nursing, and anesthesia teams. This is only possible when teams have prepared for the emergency ahead of time by running regular disaster readiness drills. In addition, the surgeon can take a few minutes to assign the specific roles and remind the team of the steps to follow in case of bleeding. This can be done right after the instruments have been introduced into the thoracic cavity and before the dissection begins.

Pressure: Pulmonary artery bleeding can be easily controlled by applying gentle pressure as it is a low-pressure system. Attempts at controlling the bleeding by applying the instrument directly to the artery should be discouraged as this tends to enlarge the tear or make the injury worse. The best approach is to have two tightly rolled sponges in the field next to the vessel being dissected. In the event of bleeding, a rolled sponge is placed over the bleeding point with a robotic instrument (usually Cadiere forceps) and pressure is maintained for at least 7 to 10 minutes if necessary. For a minor injury, this maneuver may be all is required. Next, the assistant introduces a tightly rolled sponge with "EVARREST" fibrin sealant patch on one side (Ethicon, Inc. Somerville, NJ, USA). The patch attached to a tightly rolled sponge is grasped by the other robotic instrument [26]. In a swift motion, the sponge in the hand-applying pressure is removed and replaced with the sponge carrying the EVERREST patch. The patch is held over the bleeding point with gentle pressure for 3–5 minutes. Following this, the patch should be left in place and continued pressure applied on the sponge/patch composite by the assistant instrument. The tendency to assess the injury by removing the patch should be avoided until proximal control is obtained.

It is important to emphasize that the experience of the surgeon with robotic procedures should dictate the next steps following control of the bleeding. For the less experienced surgeons, the safest strategy is to maintain pressure control of the bleeding and calmly convert to a thoracotomy.

Safe conversion to thoracotomy: A second trained surgeon is called to the room to help the primary surgeon. Once the bleeding is under control, the camera is disconnected from the robotic arm and moved to the access port for continued visualization of the pleural space and ensure there is no further bleeding. The camera port is usually near the site of the thoracotomy and needs to be removed. While gentle pressure on the roll patch is maintained with the most anterior arm, remove the posterior arms to provide room for the posterolateral thoracotomy, which should be performed calmly and under control. Performing a "crash" thoracotomy while still bleeding profusely is a losing battle that will result in a poor outcome. The chest is entered through the fifth intercostal space directly over the oblique fissure in order to have full access to the hilum and the proximal pulmonary artery. During the time that the thoracotomy is being performed, using the camera port the assistant can introduce a long metal suction to place direct pressure on the rolled sponge and/or sponge/EVERREST patch and to suction excess blood. Once the thoracotomy is performed and the ribs spread apart, a sponge stick can be introduced to apply direct pressure to the artery if necessary. The remaining robotic arms are removed, and the robot is then moved away from the operating table to allow the surgeon and the first assistant gain proximal control of the PA. Surgeons with greater experience can obtain proximal control and repair the vascular injury by robotic or endoscopic techniques. However, it must be emphasized that conversion to a thoracotomy should be seen as the safest technique and conversion should be performed in a timely fashion and not as a last resort.

Proximal control: Two types of PAI dictate the operative approach. Injury to a proximal vessel during a right or left upper lobectomy (injury to the truncus) usually requires temporary control of the bleeding by applying pressure followed by thoracotomy and vessel repair. More distal injuries to smaller branches of the PA during upper lobectomies and those during lower lobectomies can be repaired robotically by following a structured approach or by thoracotomy. For these more distal injuries, once the vessel is hemostatic, the surgeon obtains proximal control by passing a vessel loop around the pulmonary artery, double loop around it, and gently pulling up to completely stop its blood flow. At this point, the patch sponge composite is removed and the injury is repaired using 4-0 or 5-0 polypropylene suture. On occasion, a hem-o-lock can be applied robotically to the proximal site of the injury to obtain proximal control of a smaller branch of the PA. The vessel is transected and the other end is controlled with a clip.

10. Postoperative management

Patients are extubated in the operating room immediately after the operation and are transported to the recovery room. For the first 12 to 24 h, we prefer to keep the chest tube on suction to ensure lung expansion and egress of any blood or fluid. We utilize a multimodal opioid sparing protocol for pain management, which consists of oral acetaminophen, intravenous or oral NSAID's, gabapentin, and as-needed intravenous and oral narcotics medications. Patients are usually able to spend time out of bed in a chair and ambulate on postoperative day one. Standard recommendations also include deep-vein/pulmonary embolism thromboprophylaxis and incentive spirometry. In our practice, chest tubes are removed when output is less than 5 cc/kg of ideal body weight. If air leak is present or output exceeds this parameter, patients are sent home with a smaller collection device such as the Atrium Express Mini 500 dry seal as early as postoperative day 1. In most patients, this can be removed in 2–5 days. Patients are seen in follow-up in our clinic within 2 weeks to review the pathology report, ensure adequate postoperative recovery, and discuss adjuvant therapy or next steps in their treatment plan.

Author details

Raghav Chandra[1] and Alberto de Hoyos[2]*

1 Department of Surgery, University of Texas Southwestern Medical Center, Dallas, TX, United States

2 Department of Cardiothoracic Surgery, Atrium Health Wake Forest University, Winston Salem, NC, United States

*Address all correspondence to: adehoyos1957@gmail.com

References

[1] Linsky P, Wei B. Robotic lobectomy. Journal of Visualized Surgery. 2017;**3**:1-6

[2] Kim MP. Robotic lobectomy leads to excellent survival in lung cancer patients. Journal of Thoracic Disease. 2018;**10**:S3184

[3] Williamson T, Song S-E. Robotic surgery techniques to improve traditional laparoscopy. JSLS: Journal of the Society of Laparoscopic & Robotic Surgeons. 2022;**26**:1-11

[4] Ferguson JM, Pitt B, Kuntz A, et al. Comparing the accuracy of the da Vinci xi and da Vinci Si for image guidance and automation. The International Journal of Medical Robotics and Computer Assisted Surgery. 2020;**16**:1-10

[5] Inc., Intuitive. Da Vinci Surgical Systems. Available from: https://www.intuitive.com/en-us/products-and-services/da-vinci/systems

[6] Cao C, Manganas C, Ang SC, Peeceeyen S, Yan TD. Video-assisted thoracic surgery versus open thoracotomy for non-small cell lung cancer: A meta-analysis of propensity score-matched patients. Interactive Cardiovascular and Thoracic Surgery. 2013;**16**:244-249

[7] Li C, Hu Y, Huang J, et al. Comparison of robotic-assisted lobectomy with video-assisted thoracic surgery for stage IIB–IIIA non-small cell lung cancer. Translational Lung Cancer Research. 2019;**8**:820

[8] Haruki T, Takagi Y, Kubouchi Y, et al. Comparison between robot-assisted thoracoscopic surgery and video-assisted thoracoscopic surgery for mediastinal and hilar lymph node dissection in lung cancer surgery. Interactive CardioVascular and Thoracic Surgery. 2021;**33**:409-417

[9] Veronesi G, Abbas AE-S, Muriana P, et al. Perioperative outcome of robotic approach versus manual videothoracoscopic major resection in patients affected by early lung cancer: Results of a randomized multicentric study (ROMAN study). Frontiers in Oncology. 2021;**3407**:1-9

[10] Ma J, Li X, Zhao S, Wang J, Zhang W, Sun G. Robot-assisted thoracic surgery versus video-assisted thoracic surgery for lung lobectomy or segmentectomy in patients with non-small cell lung cancer: A meta-analysis. BMC Cancer. 2021;**21**:1-16

[11] NCCN. NCCN clinical practice guidelines in oncology: Non-small cell. Lung Cancer. 2022;**20**(5):1-34

[12] Veronesi G. Robotic lobectomy and segmentectomy for lung cancer: Results and operating technique. Journal of Thoracic Disease. 2015;7:S122

[13] Brunelli A, Kim AW, Berger KI, Addrizzo-Harris DJ. Physiologic evaluation of the patient with lung cancer being considered for resectional surgery: Diagnosis and management of lung cancer: American College of Chest Physicians evidence-based clinical practice guidelines. Chest. 2013;**143**:e166S-e190S

[14] Kneuertz PJ, D'Souza DM, Moffatt-Bruce SD, Merritt RE. Robotic lobectomy has the greatest benefit in patients with marginal pulmonary function. Journal of Cardiothoracic Surgery. 2018;**13**:1-7

[15] Cerfolio RJ, Bryant AS. How to teach robotic pulmonary resection. Seminars in Thoracic and Cardiovascular Surgery. 2013;**25**: Elsevier:76-82

[16] Cerfolio RJ, Watson C, Minnich DJ, Calloway S, Wei B. One hundred planned robotic segmentectomies: Early results, technical details, and preferred port placement. The Annals of Thoracic Surgery. 2016;**101**:1089-1096

[17] Balsara KR, Balderson SS, D'Amico TA. Surgical techniques to avoid parenchymal injury during lung resection (fissureless lobectomy). Thoracic surgery Clinics. 2010;**20**:365-369

[18] Decaluwé H. Video-assisted thoracic surgery tunnel technique: An alternative fissureless approach for anatomical lung resections. Video-Assisted Thoracoscopic Surgery. 2017;**2**:45-45

[19] Cerfolio RJ, Bess KM, Wei B, Minnich DJ. Incidence, results, and our current intraoperative technique to control major vascular injuries during minimally invasive robotic thoracic surgery. The Annals of Thoracic Surgery. 2016;**102**:394-399

[20] Novellis P, Jadoon M, Cariboni U, Bottoni E, Pardolesi A, Veronesi G. Management of robotic bleeding complications. Annals of Cardiothoracic Surgery. 2019;**8**:292

[21] Cao C, Cerfolio RJ, Louie BE, et al. Incidence, management, and outcomes of intraoperative catastrophes during robotic pulmonary resection. The Annals of Thoracic Surgery. 2019;**108**:1498-1504

[22] Louie BE. Catastrophes and complicated intraoperative events during robotic lung resection. Journal of Visualized Surgery. 2017;**3**:1-7

[23] Mei J, Pu Q, Liao H, Ma L, Zhu Y, Liu L. A novel method for troubleshooting vascular injury during anatomic thoracoscopic pulmonary resection without conversion to thoracotomy. Surgical Endoscopy. 2013;**27**:530-537

[24] Decaluwe H, Petersen RH, Hansen H, et al. Major intraoperative complications during video-assisted thoracoscopic anatomical lung resections: An intention-to-treat analysis. European Journal of Cardio-Thoracic Surgery. 2015;**48**:588-599

[25] Pagès P-B, Gutierrez I, Baste J-M. Pulmonary artery repair during robotic lung resection: Narrative review and management. Journal of Visualized Surgery. 2021;**8**:1-8

[26] Gharagozloo F, Meyer M. Technique of robotic lobectomy III: Control of major vascular injury, the 5 "P"'s. Mini-Invasive Surgery. 2020;**4**:57

Section 4

Sublobar Anatomic Lung Resections

Chapter 5

Segmental Resection in Early-Stage Lung Cancer

Balasubramanian Venkitaraman, Jiang Lei and Suhaildeen Kajamohideen

Abstract

The minimum standard surgical resection required for curative surgical management of carcinoma of lung had been lobectomy, established based on The Lung Cancer Study Group results, published decades earlier. Recent data show similar oncological outcomes for patients undergoing lobar and sublobar resection with proper patient selection. Randomized trials are underway to statistically establish their equivalence. Segmentectomy is a demanding procedure requiring an in-depth understanding of surgical anatomy and its variations and surgical expertise. Many techniques are described, by various specialists, to perform segmental resection, with their own advantages and shortcomings.

Keywords: segmental resection, carcinoma lung, sublobar resection, lobectomy, video-assisted thoracoscopic surgery

1. Introduction

The surgical management of lung cancer has witnessed major advances during the last 1–2 decades; most important would be the minimally invasive surgical techniques and conservatism in parenchymal resection. The lung cancer study group publication by Ginsberg et al. [1] comparing lobectomy and limited resection for early lung cancers concluded the latter to have inferior outcomes. However, this study was part of an old era where the imaging techniques were primitive and pathological understanding and classifications of lung cancer were quite different. Recent updates in the pathological classification of bronchoalveolar carcinoma have given newer terminologies: minimally invasive adenocarcinoma (MIA) and adenocarcinoma in situ (AIS), which after complete surgical resection has shown to have very good survival.

Studies by Altorki et al., Lin et al. also, have shown segmental resection for select early-stage lung cancer patients can provide good outcomes compared to lobectomy [2, 3].

2. Anatomy

The lungs are composed of functional divisions known as bronchopulmonary segments, each having its independent blood supply and air supply. The bronchi of lobes ramify and divide into divisions for the segments, which are in turn accompanied by the arteries. The venous circulation however is intersegmental and goes through the septae between the segments.

The right side lung is further divided into the right upper, middle, and lower lobes. The right upper lobe further consists of 3 segments namely:

1. S1—Apical segment

2. S2—Posterior segment

3. S3—Anterior segment

S1 is the superior most as its name suggests, posterior and inferior to it is the segment S2 and anterior to it is the segment S3. The latter two are bounded below by the horizontal fissure separating the upper and middle lobes.

The middle lobe of the right lung is divided into two segments: the lateral/costal portion—S4 and the medial/hilar—S5.

The right lower lobe of the lung consists of 5 segments:

1. S6—Superior basal segment

2. S7—Medial basal segment

3. S8—Anterior basal segment

4. S9—Lateral basal segment

5. S10—Posterior basal segment

The left lung has two lobes: the upper and lower lobes. The right upper lobe of the left lung has fewer segmental divisions compared to the right upper lobe, as few of them are merged together.

1. Apico-Posterior segment (S1 + S2)

2. Anterior segment (S3)

3. Superior lingula segment (S4)

4. Inferior lingula segment (S5)

The left lower lobe has 4 segments (one lesser compared to right lower lobe)

1. Superior basal (S6)

2. Anteromedial basal segment (S7 + S8)

3. Lateral basal segment (S9)

4. Posterior basal segment (S10)

3. Indication

Various studies have different selection criteria for patients undergoing segmental resection. Broadly this can be divided into those for primary lung lesions and those for metastatic conditions.

We recommend the following for selection of patients with primary lung cancer for segmental resection:

- Patients with early-stage lung cancer <2 cm, peripherally placed.
- Patients with respiratory compromise are not fit for lobectomy (a clearance of 2 cm is recommended).
- Peripheral nodule ≤2 cm with at least one of the following:
- Pure AIS histology
- Nodule has more than 50% ground glass appearance on CT
- Radiological surveillance confirms a doubling time(≥400 days).

Patients with metastatic tumors—with deposits in the lung—can also be candidates for segmental resection if these are centrally placed and are not ideal candidates for wedge resection.

4. Contraindications

These procedures are contraindicated in patients where surgery cannot be curative, i.e. patients with:

1. Presence of metastatic disease
2. Presence of N2/N3 mediastinal nodal disease

Previous surgeries to the ipsilateral lung are not a contraindication for segmental resection; however, presence of adhesions/fibrosis distorting the anatomy may preclude surgery.

Note: The visceral pleural invasion (VPI) noted on histology is a high-risk entity and segmental resections are not recommended in such patients.

5. Workup

All patients should be evaluated with pulmonary function tests and other routine investigations prior to surgery. A metastatic workup with whole-body FDG PET CT with an MRI brain should be performed to rule out a metastasis. Patients are admitted a day prior to the surgery. All cases are to be discussed in a multi-disciplinary tumor board prior to surgery. (As we do not have level 1 evidence for sublobar resection.)

6. Operative technique

We describe the technique of uniportal VATS segmental resection here.

Patient is intubated with an endotracheal double lumen tube to achieve lung isolation.

Patient is positioned on the table in the lateral decubitus position with the involved side exposed in its entirety, with a bridge underneath the chest, to spread out the ribs. Surgeon stands in front of the patient with assistant standing behind and the camera placed at the cranial end (**Figure 1**).

Depending on the lesion location, the uniportal utilitarian incision is placed on the 4th/5th intercostal space along the anterior axillary line (**Figure 1**). The incision is deepened and extended into the thoracic cavity, along the upper border of the rib. A wound protector/sleeve is used to cover the incision. Camera is placed in the anterior aspect of the incision and the thoracic cavity is inspected for any pleural deposits/effusion.

In lesions that are difficult to localize and deep within the parenchyma, preoperative localization techniques are helpful.

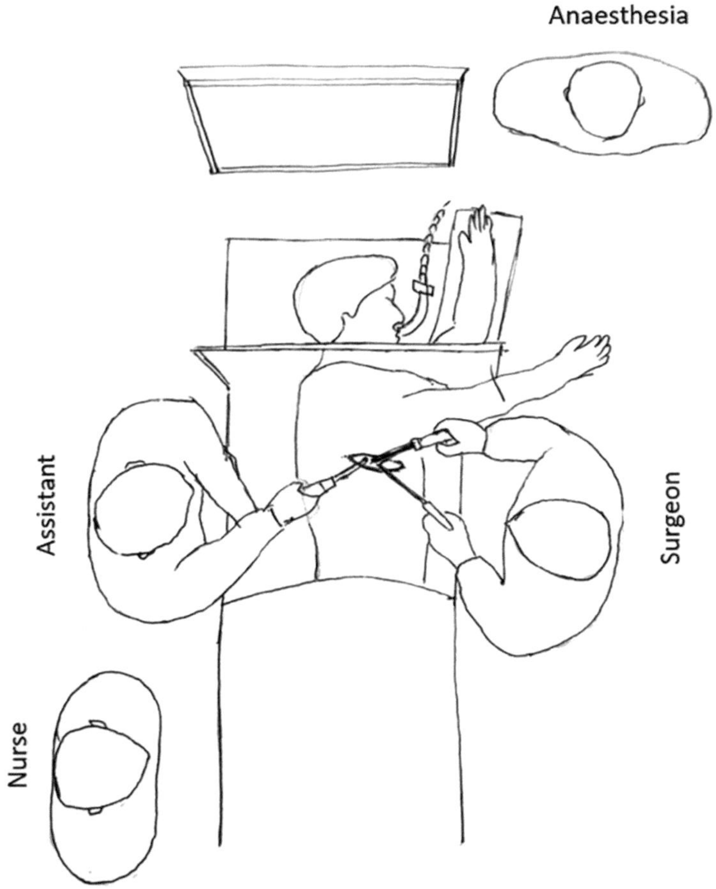

Figure 1.
Schematic representation of the operation theater set up for uniportal thoracoscopic surgery. Uniportal incision on the lateral aspect of the ipsilateral chest wall. Surgeon standing anteriorly, assistant standing behind the patient, monitor placed on the head end aspect.

- Three-dimensional reconstruction and spatial orientation [4]
- CT guided wire placement/needloscopic [5, 6]
- Intraoperative imaging—radiograph/ultrasound
- Finger palpation

Once the segment to be removed is localized, further dissection takes place along the bronchus/artery and the branch leading to the segment is dissected out. Different techniques can be used for identification of the intersegmental plane during the procedure. These include the conventional deflation-inflation technique, where the bronchial division is divided and the rest of the lung is inflated. The deflated parenchymal markings provide us with the intersegmental plane or the plane for parenchymal division. However, there could be other communications that may cross-inflate the segment to be divided, giving a wrong plane of resection.

Another way is the inflation-deflation technique, where the lung is inflated and the bronchus to segment is divided and the lung is deflated [7]. Here since the bronchus is stapled, the segment remains inflated and forms the margins, helping in identifying a plane of resection. Disadvantages of this are the inflated lung many times obscures the vision and makes it difficult to apply staplers. Indocyanine green fluorescence has also been used in identification of the intersegmental plane. After the segmental artery was divided, an intravenous systemic injection of indocyanine green was given and with infrared assistance, margins were made out [8].

We use a SAFE technique for identification of the intersegmental plane, published earlier [9]. After identification and division of the segmental artery, the bronchus is identified. A small incision is made in the bronchial division of the

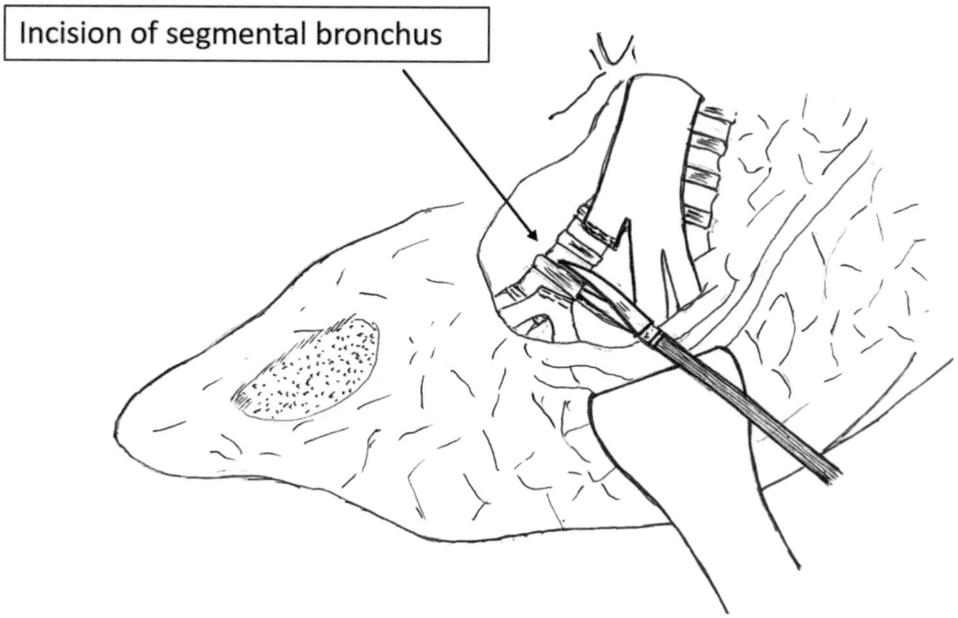

Figure 2.
Segmental bronchus being identified and an incision made with sharp scissors.

segment (**Figure 2**) and a deep vein catheter is placed into the incision directed distally into the segment to be removed (**Figure 3**). Incision on the bronchus is just enough to admit the catheter. Clamp is applied on the bronchus as shown in **Figure 4** and air is insufflated through a syringe, and the parenchyma gets inflated, defining the segmental boundary.

Once this is defined, the catheter is removed and the segmental bronchus divided using endostaplers and the distal cut end is lifted up. Parenchymal dissection is done further to aid in the placement of the staplers for division of the parenchyma. Once parenchymal division takes place, we check for air leak.

Nodal dissection needs to be performed in patients with invasive lung cancer according to the AJCC /IASLC station map, removing the level 1 and level 2 nodes – as per the location of the tumor.

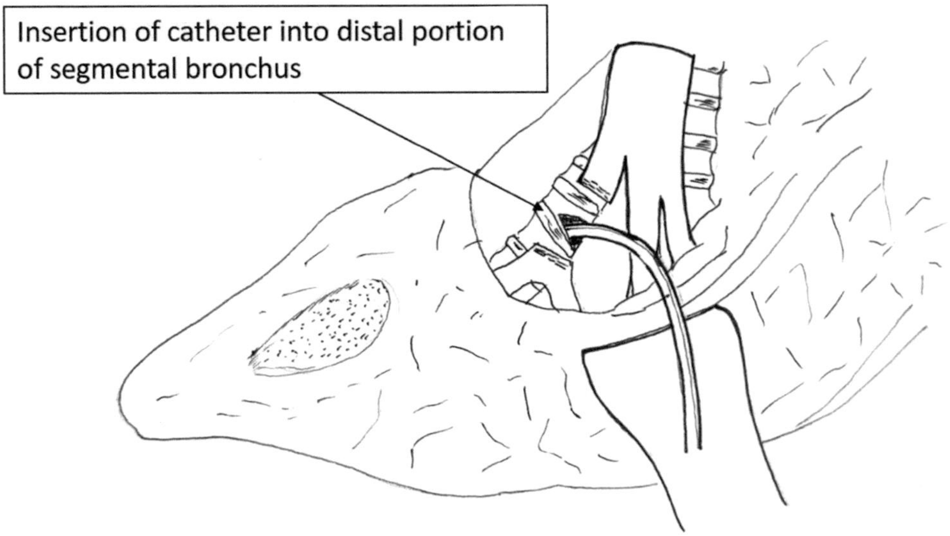

Figure 3.
Deep vein catheter placed through the incision, directed distally into the segmental bronchus.

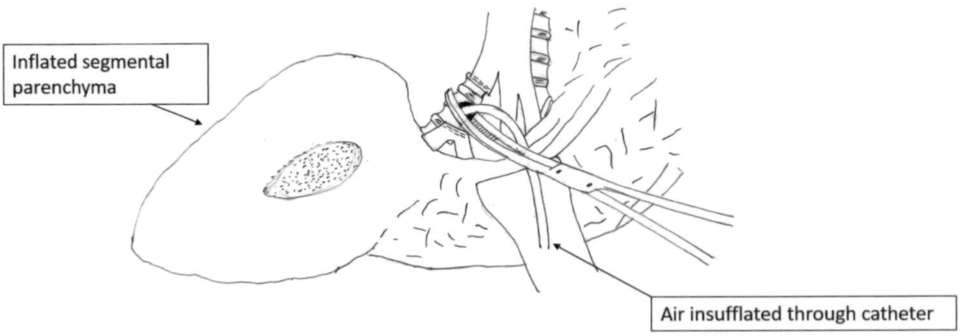

Figure 4.
Air insufflated through the catheter, showing inflation of the segmental parenchyma. This helps in parenchymal demarcation, helping to identify the intersegmental plane for division.

7. Commonly performed segmental resections: technique

7.1 Left side: lingulectomy (S4-S5)

After approaching the hilum thoracoscopically, from anteriorly, the left superior pulmonary vein is identified and traced to identify the lingula branch. This is divided with staplers to reveal the bronchial anatomy. The upper lobe bronchial division and the lingular divisions are identified, the latter is divided with staplers, after defining the intersegmental plane. The lingualar artery is acceptable is approached as the visaulised, better posteriorly, and divided, followed by parenchymal division.

7.2 Left upper lobectomy: lingula sparing (S1-S3)

The left hemithorax is approached thoracoscopically and in an anterior approach, the hilar structures are identified. The left superior pulmonary vein is identified and dissected out to identify the branches to the upper lobe. Branches are divided with staplers and then the bronchial tree is visualized. The same is dissected out to identify the S1, S2, and S3 branches which are then divided with staplers.

The left upper lobe receives short segmental arterial branches from the left main pulmonary artery as it winds around the hilum, going posteriorly. These are dissected and taken individually if needed and then the parenchymal transection is made.

7.3 Superior segmentectomy: lower lobe (S6): both sides

On either side, the inferior pulmonary ligament is dissected out and the inferior pulmonary vein is identified. From a posterior approach, the superior segmental vein S6 is identified in the fissure and is divided, preserving the basilar branches. The S6 arterial branch can be identified posteriorly and divided. The lower lobe bronchus can be traced and the S6 origin identified, cut, and catheter placement is done. S6 is inflated and parenchymal margins are marked out. S6 is then divided with staplers and parenchymal transection is completed.

7.4 Basilar segmentectomy: S7-S10

Similar to the superior segmentectomy approach, the inferior pulmonary vein is first identified and then dissected out to identify the S6 branch. The vein distal to this is divided. Inferior pulmonary artery distal to the S6 branch is divided, better in the posterior approach. The lower lobe bronchus is traced and the division distal to the S6 branch is canulated and the parenchyma is inflated. The bronchus is divided and then parenchymal division is done.

8. Node dissection

Systematic nodal dissection and systematic nodal sampling both have been proved to have similar outcomes, especially in patients with N0 on imaging [10]. Nodal dissection should be based on the lesion location.

A minimum of 3—N2 level nodes should be sampled with a total of at least 6 nodes.

For left upper—left levels 4, 5, 6, and subcarinal should be removed along with hilar node dissection.

For left lower lobe lesions—left levels 7, 8, 9, and 10 should be removed along with hilar node dissection.

For right upper lobe lesions—right level 2.4.7 with hilar nodes need to be removed.

For right lower lobe lesions—right levels 7, 8, 9, and 10 with hilar nodes need to be removed.

9. Conclusion

Segmental resection is a sound alternative to lobar resection in select patients with early-stage lung cancer. Proper selection of patients becomes an important component to ensure good outcomes. A nodal dissection needs to be accompanied by segmental resection in patients with preoperative diagnosis of invasive primary lung cancer. In patients with uncertain pathologies, an intraoperative frozen section is recommended to help in completing nodal dissection for malignant conditions. Larger trials are underway and their results can confirm or refute the oncological safety of segmentectomy in early-stage lung cancer [11].

Conflict of interest

The authors declare no conflict of interest.

Author details

Balasubramanian Venkitaraman[1*], Jiang Lei[2] and Suhaildeen Kajamohideen[1]

1 Division of Thoracic Oncology, Department of Surgical Oncology, Sri Ramachandra Institute of Higher Education and Research, Chennai, India

2 Department of Thoracic Surgery, Shanghai Pulmonary Hospital, Shanghai, People's Republic of China

*Address all correspondence to: bala.oncosurg@gmail.com

References

[1] Ginsberg RJ, Rubinstein LV. Randomized trial of lobectomy versus limited resection for T1 N0 non-small cell lung cancer. Lung Cancer Study Group. The Annals of Thoracic Surgery. 1995;**60**(3):615-622; discussion 622-623

[2] Altorki NK, Yip R, Hanaoka T, Bauer T, Aye R, Kohman L, et al. Sublobar resection is equivalent to lobectomy for clinical stage 1A lung cancer in solid nodules. The Journal of Thoracic and Cardiovascular Surgery. 2014;**147**(2):754-762; discussion 762-764

[3] Lin YJ, Chiang XH, Lu TP, Hsieh MS, Lin MW, Hsu HH, et al. Thoracoscopic lobectomy versus sublobar resection for pStage I geriatric non-small cell lung cancer. Frontiers in Oncology. 2021;**11**:777590

[4] Xu G, Chen C, Zheng W, Zhu Y, Chen H, Cai B. Application of the IQQA-3D imaging interpretation and analysis system in uniportal video-assisted thoracoscopic anatomical segmentectomy: A series study. Journal of Thoracic Disease. 2019;**11**(5):2058-2066

[5] Yang SM, Wu WT, Liu YH, Ko HJ. Needlescopic-assisted uniportal video-assisted thoracoscopic pulmonary anatomical segmentectomy. Journal of Visualized Surgery. 2017;**3**:138

[6] Duan L, Jiang G, Yang Y. One hundred and fifty-six cases of anatomical pulmonary segmentectomy by uniportal video-assisted thoracic surgery: A 2-year learning experience. European Journal of Cardio-Thoracic Surgery: Official Journal of the European Association for Cardio-thoracic Surgery. 2018;**54**(4):677-682

[7] Han KN, Kim HK, Choi YH. Comparison of single port versus multiport thoracoscopic segmentectomy. Journal of Thoracic Disease. 2016;**8**(Suppl 3):S279-S286

[8] Mun M, Okumura S, Nakao M, Matsuura Y, Nakagawa K. Indocyanine green fluorescence-navigated thoracoscopic anatomical segmentectomy. Journal of Visualized Surgery. 2017;**3**:80

[9] Venkitaraman. Video-assisted uniportal pulmonary segmentectomy: Description of Safe Accurate Feasible and Easy technique and analysis of short-term outcome. Video-Assisted Thoracic Surgery. 2020;**5**:2. Available from: https://vats.amegroups.com/article/view/5804/html

[10] Darling GE, Allen MS, Decker PA, Ballman K, Malthaner RA, Inculet RI, et al. Randomized trial of mediastinal lymph node sampling versus complete lymphadenectomy during pulmonary resection in the patient with N0 or N1 (less than hilar) non-small cell carcinoma: Results of the American college of surgery oncology group Z0030 trial. The Journal of Thoracic and Cardiovascular Surgery. 2011;**141**(3):662-670

[11] Altorki NK, Wang X, Wigle D, Gu L, Darling G, Ashrafi AS, et al. Perioperative mortality and morbidity after sublobar versus lobar resection for early-stage non-small-cell lung cancer: Post-hoc analysis of an international, randomised, phase 3 trial (CALGB/Alliance 140503). The Lancet Respiratory Medicine. 2018;**6**(12):915-924

Section 5

Intensive Care Unit Management after Lobectomy

Chapter 6

Intensive Care Unit Management after Pulmonary Lobectomy

Naveen Yadav and Sankalp Purwar

Abstract

The patients with pulmonary lobectomy invariably are shifted to the intensive care unit/high-dependency unit after the surgery because these patients can have significant minor and major complications. These complications following pulmonary lobectomy are preventable, and early identification in ICU can lead to reduced morbidity and mortality. Good intensive care management after pulmonary lobectomy can reduce the cost by decreasing the number of days patient stays in the hospital. This chapter will broadly discuss the common complications encountered in ICU after pulmonary lobectomy and approach to manage them.

Keywords: pulmonary lobectomy, postoperative complication, postoperative pain control

1. Introduction

Lobectomy is removal of an individual lobe by ligating its contributing pulmonary artery, pulmonary vein, and lobar bronchi. Indications for pulmonary lobectomy include malignancy, to diagnose pathology of a nodule or mass, traumatic injury, broncho-pleural fistula, and bronchiectasis.

2. Surgical technique

Detailed surgical techniques are beyond the realm of this chapter and have been explained in other chapters. Broadly speaking, it is open or minimally invasive lung resection. Minimally invasive techniques have shown benefit when compared with open thoracotomy. Several systematic reviews have reported faster recovery and shorter hospital stay with minimally invasive technique [1–7]. Older patients are independent sooner with minimally invasive procedures compared with larger chest incisions despite the extent of surgery being similar internally.

3. Selection of the patients at risk after pulmonary lobectomy for ICU admission

The post-operative mortality rates after a major thoracic surgical procedure can range from 2 to 5%. The cardiopulmonary morbidity can range between 20 to 40%

and this can result in prolonged hospital stay and increased cost. There are several patients related and procedure related risk factors which can indicate a high risk of postoperative complications.

The patient related risk factors include:

1. ASA (American Society of Anaesthesiologists) physical status ≥ 3

2. S-MPM (Surgical mortality probability model) ≥ 6 points

3. RCRI (Revised cardiac risk index) > 2 points

4. ThRCRI (Thoracic RCRI) >1.5 points

5. ARISCAT (Assess Respiratory Risk in Surgical patients in Catalonia risk index) > 45 points

6. Preoperative FEV1< 60%

7. Predictive-DLCO < 30%

The Procedure-related risk factors include:

1. High risk procedure

2. Major intraoperative complications like refractory hypotension, myocardial ischemia, cardiac arrhythmia, major haemorrhage, and bronchial aspiration

3. Low level of hospital and operative expertise

4. Emergency operation

It is usually advisable to shift any of the above patients to ICU for post-operative monitoring.

4. ICU management

4.1 Bronchial hygiene

While patient is intubated, regular suctioning is helpful for secretion clearance, avoid lung collapse and development of pneumonia. After extubation, chest physiotherapy, incentive spirometry and ambulation are important to promote secretion clearance.

4.2 Ventilation

Usually, patients are extubated in theatre or recovery post operatively. If they continue to be ventilated, aim is to minimize barotrauma by using low tidal volume ventilation and moderate levels of PEEP (less than 10 cm water). Significant air trapping and auto-PEEP is not uncommon in patients with emphysema. Adequate tidal volume and expiratory time and avoiding excess PEEP will help in preventing air trapping. Ventilator should be weaned as soon as possible to prevent nosocomial infection and promote patient participation in early mobilisation and physiotherapy.

In selected patients, high-flow nasal cannula oxygen therapy may be used cautiously to treat hypoxemia after extubation in the early postoperative period [8]. While not routinely used after pulmonary resection, continuous positive airway pressure (CPAP) is reasonable if otherwise indicated (e.g., obstructive sleep apnoea). In small studies, CPAP appears to improve oxygenation without increasing air leakage through the chest drain or the incidence of other postoperative complications [9, 10].

4.3 Hemodynamics and fluid management

It is important to maintain adequate intravascular volume to maintain adequate cardiac output. Fluid therapy is aimed at maintaining low or low-normal cardiac filling pressures. Restrictive fluid strategy may reduce pulmonary complications and facilitate early extubation. While the fluid regimen should be individualized to optimize cardiac output and oxygen delivery, excessive fluid administration (i.e., >3 L in the 24 hours of the perioperative period) is associated with acute lung injury and delayed recovery after open thoracic surgery [11–17]. In one study, the risk of acute lung injury increased for each 500 mL increment of perioperative fluid (odds ratio [OR] 1.17, 95% CI 1.00–1.36) [12].

Invasive cardiac monitoring is usually not needed beyond first 24 hours. In our practice, we prefer to give bolus dose of intravenous fluids rather than continuous maintenance fluid.

4.4 Vasopressors

The combination of general anaesthesia and thoracic epidural analgesia can cause hypotension. Rather than administering additional fluid to support BP in a euvolemic patient, we suggest using an infusion of a low dose of a vasopressor agent typically noradrenaline to maintain adequate Mean Arterial Pressure.

4.5 Post-operative analgesia

Thoracotomy induces severe postoperative pain which can cause respiratory complications, such as hypoxia, atelectasis, and pulmonary infections. In addition, inadequate pain control can lead to post-thoracotomy pain syndrome, which may continue for many years; therefore excellent analgesia after lung surgery is vital. This will allow deep breathing, coughing and early mobilisation.

It is well established that VATS offers the benefit of major pulmonary resection with decreased early postoperative pain, decreased need for opioid analgesia, decreased hospital stay, and faster recovery and return to preoperative activities [18, 19]. Minimally invasive lung resection confers an improved short-term quality of life and decreased chronic pain as documented in several studies [20–23].

Guidelines on postoperative analgesia published by the American Society of Regional Analgesia and Pain Medicine and the American Society of Anaesthesiologists' Committee on Regional Anaesthesia emphasise the importance of multimodal agents which work on different pain pathways and use of systemic and local-regional analgesia to support opioid-sparing strategies and reduce systemic side effects.

4.5.1 Opioids

Administration routes are multiple including intravenous, subcutaneous, and oral preparations. The most habitual way is the patient-controlled analgesia (PCA) transitioning to oral opioids once patient has resumed oral intake. Common agents for PCA are morphine, fentanyl, and oxycodone. Other common opioids are codeine and tramadol. Basal infusion of opioids, with or without PCA, must be limited in opioid-naive patients because of the increased risk of side effects, including hypotension, respiratory depression, itching, nausea, vomiting, ileus, confusion, and sedation.

4.5.2 Opioid sparing agents

With Non-steroidal anti-inflammatory drugs (NSAIDs) the use of opioids is reduced but more risk of kidney injury, gastric bleeding, and effect on platelets aggregation. In our practice, nonsteroidal drugs are usually avoided if concomitant pleurodesis is performed. Paracetamol is an acetanilide derivative which can be given both orally and intravenously. Paracetamol acts by inhibiting substance P action and central prostaglandin synthesis. N-methyl-D-aspartate (NMDA) antagonists Ketamine is another opioid sparing agent, but side effects include hallucinations and restricted mobility with continuous intravenous infusion. Gabapentinoids may help reducing neuropathic pain after thoracic surgery. Literature indicates that preoperative administration of gabapentinoids may also reduce postoperative pain and opioid usage.

4.5.3 Regional analgesia

Thoracic epidural analgesia (TEA) is considered the gold standard technique in pain management, usually recommended as first line after thoracic surgery. It provides better pain relief than opioid PCA treatment and permits a faster recovery. Local anaesthetics added to opioids in TEA increase analgesia efficacy. Major deterrent to epidural use is its invasiveness. Other side effects could be sympathetic blockade, respiratory depression, and urinary retention.

Thoracic paravertebral block (TPVB) is commonly used, especially with VATS approach. It is often proposed as an alternative to TEA because results in term of pain control are comparable to TEA, with fewer side effects. Pain in the very immediate post-operative period can be covered with a single shot of TPVB but to have a longer analgesic effect, a continuous TPVB analgesia with a catheter placed in the paravertebral space should be considered.

Intercostal nerve block is a very well-known technique, especially to treat pain after thoracotomy. Both the single-shot technique and the continuous infusion are possible with infusion more effective after thoracic surgery. The continuous infusion of local anaesthetic in the intercostal space provides pain relief comparable to TEA, until approximately the 5th postoperative days after open surgery.

Serratus anterior plane block (SAPB) is a thoracic wall nerve block that covers the lateral cutaneous branch of the intercostal nerves from T2 to T9. The SAPB provides more hemodynamic stability compared with TEA after thoracotomy and reinforces PCA analgesia reducing pain and opioid use. In patients undergoing VATS, the locoregional techniques help in both reducing pain and opioid consumption in the first 24–48 hours after intervention.

4.6 Antibiotic prophylaxis

Postoperative antibiotic prophylaxis after lobectomy is controversial. Deguchi et al has shown that prophylactic antibiotic administration in both intraoperative and postoperative periods reduced the incidence of pneumonia after pulmonary lobectomy for non-small cell lung cancer [24]. A prospective randomized double-blind trial of flash cefuroxime versus forty-eight- hour cefuroxime in pulmonary surgery has shown the benefit of reducing the rate of deep infections and particularly the rate of empyema [25]. However, a double blind, placebo controlled, randomized trial by Oxman et al has shown not to reduce the number of infectious complications compared with preoperative prophylaxis only [26]. In our institution, 24 hours of antibiotic post operatively is usually prescribed based on local microbiologic susceptibility.

4.7 Nutrition

Early introduction of nutrition helps in recovery post operatively. Inadequate calorie and protein intake during critical illness is associated with poor clinical outcomes. Nutritional risk screening should be performed within 24–48 hours of hospital admission to identify patients at high risk of malnutrition. Nutrition Risk in the Critically Ill (NUTRIC score) and Nutritional Risk Screening 2002 (NRS 2002) have been extensively studied as screening tools. Once a patient is identified as at risk, formal nutritional assessment by a trained healthcare professional should be performed. An enteral formula with appropriate macronutrient and micronutrient composition may assist patients in meeting nutritional goals. Conventionally, enteral nutrition is encouraged to help maintain gut structure and function including that of the T-cell associated lymphoid tissues and neutrophil activation [27]. The ASPEN guidelines published recently suggest feeding between 12 and 25 kcal/kg in the first 7–10 days of ICU stay with protein intake 1.2–2 kcal/kg/day [28]. Parenteral nutrition is usually not needed in postoperative patients with pulmonary lobectomy. However, if enteral feed is not tolerated, parenteral nutrition may be considered.

4.8 Renal failure

Incidence of acute kidney injury has been reported in 6–10% patients undergoing lung resection surgery with more complicated intra-hospital course. Hence, maintain normovolemia, normal cardiac output, avoid nephrotoxic medications and monitor urine output along with renal function.

4.9 Enhanced recovery protocols

These typically incorporate aspects of preoperative, intraoperative, and postoperative care to reduce morbidity. Specific Enhanced Recovery Protocols for thoracic surgery have shown benefits in reduced opioid use, less fluid administration, decreased pulmonary and cardiac morbidity, and reduced hospital length of stay [29–31].

5. Chest tube management

Following lobectomy, one or more chest tubes are placed in the thoracic cavity. Chest tubes are typically placed through a separate incision when a thoracotomy is performed. When a minimally invasive technique is performed, chest tubes can also be placed directly through the port sites. In a trial that randomly assigned 40 patients to thoracic drainage using the same intercostal space as the thoracotomy incision or traditional chest drainage using a separate incision, the mean lengths of hospital or intensive care unit stay, pain scores, and complications (including infection) were similar between the groups [32].

Postoperative management of chest tubes is directed by postoperative imaging, presence or absence of air leak and the volume and/or character of drainage. Following both open and minimally invasive techniques, typically the chest tube is connected to suction in the immediate postoperative period for at least 12 hours, then disconnect the suction leaving the chest tube to water seal.

The decision to place a chest tube to suction versus water seal alone, if a postoperative pleural leak is present, is controversial. Multiple randomized trials have compared outcomes for patients assigned to chest tubes placed to water seal or to suction following lung resection following a brief period of suction [33–38]. A meta-analysis that included 7 RCTs found no difference in duration of air leak, incidence of prolonged air leak, duration of chest tubes and duration of hospital stay when chest tubes were placed to suction rather than water seal [39].

Chest tubes must be evaluated multiple times every day to ensure patency of the tubes, and to assess for their on-going requirement. We leave the chest tubes in position as long as there is any air leak, or the draining fluid effluent volume is >300 mL/day.

6. Complications associated with pulmonary lobectomy in ICU

Pulmonary complications following thoracic surgery are the most common cause of morbidity followed by cardiovascular-related morbidity, and the incidence of these complications increase with increasing age. In general, complications related to minimally invasive thoracic procedures are similar to those of the open surgical approaches. Common complications following lung resection include arrhythmias, postoperative atelectasis, respiratory failure, bleeding, surgical site infection, prolonged postoperative air leak, and bronchopleural fistula.

6.1 Respiratory failure

In a secondary analysis of the American College of Surgeons Oncology Group (ACOSOG) Z0030 trial [40], the incidence of respiratory failure requiring ventilation was 3.7% and Adult Respiratory Distress Syndrome was 0.3%. Pulmonary complications such as atelectasis, bronchospasm and pneumonia can lead to respiratory failure. In a retrospective study of nearly 17,000 patients undergoing lung resection surgery, 3.5% required re-intubation. Risk factors for reintubation included age, male gender, clinically significant comorbidities (or ASA physical status ≥4), tobacco use, and prolonged duration of surgery [41].

Pulmonary oedema can be seen in 1–5% patients after pulmonary lobectomy. It is a noncardiogenic and non-infectious pulmonary oedema caused by increased permeability and diffuse alveolar damage. The treatment of this pulmonary oedema is to "keep the patient dry", early reintubation or trial of non-invasive ventilation in cases of respiratory failure. In addition, administration of inotropic/vasopressor drugs, while restricting fluid intake as mentioned above.

6.2 Cardiac arrhythmias

Supraventricular tachyarrhythmia is more common than ventricular rhythm disturbances after noncardiac thoracic surgery. Atrial fibrillation (AF) is the most common arrhythmia occurring in 10–20% of patients after lobectomy and occurs most commonly in first four days postoperatively. Risk factors for AF after lung cancer surgery are increasing age, increasing extent of operation, male sex, non-black race and stage II or greater tumour [42].

Extensive guidelines are available from the American Association for Thoracic Surgery [43]. There are some prevention strategies which help reduce the postoperative atrial fibrillation. These strategies include correction of magnesium when abnormal and also avoiding beta-blockade withdrawal for those chronically on these medications. It may be reasonable to administer diltiazem to patients with preserved cardiac function who are not on beta blockers preoperatively or to give post-operative amiodarone to reduce incidence of post-operative AF. Simple treatment strategies to control AF includes the optimization of fluid balance, correct electrolytes and treat triggering factors (bleeding, pulmonary embolism, pneumothorax, pericardial processes, airway issues, myocardial ischemia, or infection). For hemodynamically unstable patient with the new onset post-operative AF of less than 48 hours duration, emergency DC cardioversion is indicated. For hemodynamically stable patient, rate control strategy is reasonable. Agents commonly used are beta blockers, non-dihydropyridine calcium channel blockers or digoxin. Rhythm control with antiarrhythmic drugs and/or DC cardioversion can be useful for patients with hemodynamically stable new onset AF who have recurrent or refractory AF, continued symptoms, intolerance to rate control medications, or ventricular rates that cannot be adequately controlled. For rhythm control, amiodarone is the most common drug used. Other agents which can be used are sotalol and flecainide.

6.3 Haemorrhage

Post lobectomy haemorrhage is rare but most common indication for reoperation. In a recent single centre retrospective review [44], out of 1960 lobectomies, haemorrhage occurred in 2.1% cases, leading to reoperation in 1.4% and non-operative management in 0.8% cases. The median time for reoperation was 17 hours.

6.4 Postoperative leak

Persistent postoperative air leak, defined arbitrarily as pulmonary leak of more than seven days, occurs in 10–15% of patients following lobectomy. Persistent air leaks are more common in patients with severe COPD. Management is often conservative with on-going chest tube drainage or home discharge with one way flutter valve. Most air leaks seal within two weeks with conservative care. Postoperatively, patients should be extubated as soon as possible to reduce intrapulmonary pressure. Other treatments including injection of talc, other sclerosing agents and autologous blood may be helpful to close a persisting air leak. In more difficult cases, intrabronchial valves have been proposed to close alveolar pleural fistulas.

6.5 Bronchopleural fistula

Bronchopleural fistula, which is a direct communication of the bronchus and the pleural space, is a major complication of lung resection and occurs in 1–2% of lobectomies. Management requires reoperation for bronchial closure, pleural space drainage, and sterilization.

6.6 Injury to the organs

Injury to the diaphragm, liver, or spleen may occur, particularly during port placement with consequent morbidity.

7. Conclusion

ICU management of patients with pulmonary lobectomy is required for two main reasons: post-operative setting or acute complications following surgery. Careful pre-operative assessment of patients is mandatory to reduce post-operative morbidity and mortality. The requirement of ICU depends upon the patient and on local specifics. Several cardiac and respiratory complications can happen in ICU following admission after pulmonary lobectomy. Prevention and early recognition, as well as interdisciplinary cooperation are essential to obtain the best patient centred outcome.

Author details

Naveen Yadav[1*] and Sankalp Purwar[2]

1 Royal Prince Alfred Hospital, NSW, Australia

2 Flinders Medical Centre, South Australia, Australia

*Address all correspondence to: naveen.dv2@gmail.com

References

[1] Redden MD, Chin TY, van Driel ML. Surgical versus non-surgical management for pleural empyema. Cochrane Database of Systematic Reviews. 2017;**3**(3):CD010651

[2] Zhang W, Wei Y, Jiang H, et al. Video-assisted thoracoscopic surgery versus thoracotomy lymph node dissection in clinical stage I lung cancer: A meta-analysis and system review. The Annals of Thoracic Surgery. 2016;**101**:2417

[3] Meng D, Fu L, Wang L, et al. Video-assisted thoracoscopic surgery versus open thoracotomy in pulmonary metastasectomy: A meta-analysis of observational studies. Interactive Cardiovascular and Thoracic Surgery. 2016;**22**:200

[4] Cai YX, Fu XN, Xu QZ, et al. Thoracoscopic lobectomy versus open lobectomy in stage I non-small cell lung cancer: A meta-analysis. PLoS One. 2013;**8**:e82366

[5] Demmy TL, Plante AJ, Nwogu CE, et al. Discharge independence with minimally invasive lobectomy. American Journal of Surgery. 2004;**188**:698

[6] Villamizar NR, Darrabie MD, Burfeind WR, et al. Thoracoscopic lobectomy is associated with lower morbidity compared with thoracotomy. The Journal of Thoracic and Cardiovascular Surgery. 2009;**138**:419

[7] Paul S, Altorki NK, Sheng S, et al. Thoracoscopic lobectomy is associated with lower morbidity than open lobectomy: A propensity-matched analysis from the STS database. The Journal of Thoracic and Cardiovascular Surgery. 2010;**139**:366

[8] Wittenstein J, Ball L, Pelosi P, de Gama M. High-flow nasal cannula oxygen therapy in patients undergoing thoracic surgery: Current evidence and practice. Current Opinion in Anaesthesiology. 2019;**32**:44

[9] Roceto Ldos S, Galhardo FD, Saad IA, Toro IF. Continuous positive airway pressure (CPAP) after lung resection: A randomized clinical trial. São Paulo Medical Journal. 2014;**132**:41

[10] Barbagallo M, Ortu A, Spadini E, Salvadori A, Ampollini L, Internullo E, et al. Prophylactic use of helmet CPAP after pulmonary lobectomy: A prospective randomized controlled study. Respiratory Care. 2012;**57**(9):1418

[11] Licker M, de Perrot M, Spiliopoulos A, et al. Risk factors for acute lung injury after thoracic surgery for lung cancer. Anesthesia and Analgesia. 2003;**97**:1558

[12] Alam N, Park BJ, Wilton A, et al. Incidence and risk factors for lung injury after lung cancer resection. The Annals of Thoracic Surgery. 2007;**84**:1085

[13] Yao S, Mao T, Fang W, et al. Incidence and risk factors for acute lung injury after open thoracotomy for thoracic diseases. Journal of Thoracic Disease. 2013;**5**:455

[14] Licker M, Fauconnet P, Villiger Y, Tschopp JM. Acute lung injury and outcomes after thoracic surgery. Current Opinion in Anaesthesiology. 2009;**22**:61

[15] Della Rocca G, Coccia C. Acute lung injury in thoracic surgery. Current Opinion in Anaesthesiology. 2013;**26**:40

[16] Assaad S, Popescu W, Perrino A. Fluid management in thoracic surgery. Current Opinion in Anaesthesiology. 2013;**26**:31

[17] Arslantas MK, Kara HV, Tuncer BB, et al. Effect of the amount of intraoperative fluid administration on postoperative pulmonary complications following anatomic lung resections. The Journal of Thoracic and Cardiovascular Surgery. 2015;**149**:314

[18] Kirby TJ, Mack MJ, Landreneau RJ, Rice TW. Lobectomy-video-assisted thoracic surgery versus muscle-sparing thoracotomy. A randomized trial. Journal of Thoracic Cardiovascular Surgery. 1995;**109**:997

[19] Darr C, Cheufou D, Weinreich G, et al. Robotic thoracic surgery results in shorter hospital stay and lower postoperative pain compared to open thoracotomy: A matched pairs analysis. Surgical Endoscopy. 2017;**31**:4126

[20] Dales RE, Bélanger R, Shamji FM, et al. Quality-of-life following thoracotomy for lung cancer. Journal of Clinical Epidemiology. 1994;**47**:1443

[21] Li WW, Lee TW, Lam SS, et al. Quality of life following lung cancer resection: Video-assisted thoracic surgery vs thoracotomy. Chest. 2002;**122**:584

[22] Hopkins KG, Ferson PF, Shende MR, et al. Prospective study of quality of life after lung cancer resection. Annals of Translational Medicine. 2017;**5**:204

[23] Bendixen M, Jørgensen OD, Kronborg C, et al. Postoperative pain and quality of life after lobectomy via video-assisted thoracoscopic surgery or anterolateral thoracotomy for early-stage lung cancer: A randomised controlled trial. The Lancet Oncology. 2016;**17**:836

[24] Deguchi H, Tomoyasu M, Kaneko W, et al. Influence of prophylactic antibiotic duration on postoperative pneumonia following pulmonary lobectomy for non-small cell lung cancer. Journal of Thoracic Disease. 2019 Apr;**11**(4):1155-1164

[25] Bernard A, Pillet M, Goudet P, et al. Antibiotic prophylaxis in Pulmonary surgery:A prospective randomized double-blind trial of flash cefuroxime versus forty-eight -hour cefuroxime. The Journal of Thoracic and Cardiovascular Surgery. 1994;**107**:896-900

[26] Oxman D, Issa N, Marty F, et al. Postoperative antibacterial prophylaxis for the prevention of infectious complications associated with tube thoracostomy in patients undergoing elective general thoracic surgery: A double-blind, placebo -controlled, randomized trial. JAMA Surgery. 2013;**148**(5):440-446

[27] Groos S, Hunefeld G, Luciano L. Parenteral verus eneteral nutrition: Morphological changes in human adult intestinal mucosa. Journal of Submicroscopic Cytology and Pathology. 1996;**28**:61-74

[28] Compher C, Bingham AL, McCall M, et al. Guidelines for the provision of nutrition support therapy in the adult critically ill patient: The American Society for Parenteral and Enteral Nutrition. Journal of Parenteral and Enteral Nutrition. 2022;**46**:12-41

[29] Madani A, Fiore JF Jr, Wang Y, et al. An enhanced recovery pathway reduces duration of stay and complications after open pulmonary lobectomy. Surgery. 2015;**158**:899

[30] Van Haren RM, Mehran RJ, Mena GE, et al. Enhanced recovery decreases pulmonary and cardiac

complications after thoracotomy for lung cancer. The Annals of Thoracic Surgery. 2018;**106**:272

[31] Li S, Zhou K, Che G, et al. Enhanced recovery programs in lung cancer surgery: Systematic review and meta-analysis of randomized controlled trials. Cancer Management and Research. 2017;**9**:657

[32] Bachichi TG, Leão LEV, Perfeito JAJ, Miotto A, Holanda CS, Costa ADS Jr. Traditional chest drainage versus drainage by thoracotomy: A prospective randomized study. Einstein (Sao Paulo). 2020;**18**:eAO4409

[33] Marshall MB, Deeb ME, Bleier JI, et al. Suction vs water seal after pulmonary resection: A randomized prospective study. Chest. 2002;**121**:831

[34] Ayed AK. Suction versus water seal after thoracoscopy for primary spontaneous pneumothorax: Prospective randomized study. The Annals of Thoracic Surgery. 2003;**75**:1593

[35] Leo F, Duranti L, Girelli L, et al. Does external pleural suction reduce prolonged air leak after lung resection? Results from the Air INTrial after 500 randomized cases. The Annals of Thoracic Surgery. 2013;**96**:1234

[36] Cerfolio RJ, Bass C, Katholi CR. Prospective randomized trial compares suction versus water seal for air leaks. The Annals of Thoracic Surgery. 2001;**71**:1613

[37] Alphonso N, Tan C, Utley M, et al. A prospective randomized controlled trial of suction versus non-suction to the under-water seal drains following lung resection. European Journal of Cardio-Thoracic Surgery. 2005;**27**:391

[38] Gocyk W, Kużdżał J, Włodarczyk J, et al. comparison of suction versus nonsuction drainage after lung resections: A Prospective Randomized Trial. The Annals of Thoracic Surgery. 2016;**102**:1119

[39] Coughlin SM, Emmerton-Coughlin HMA, Malthaner R. Management of chest tubes after pulmonary resection: A systematic review and meta-analysis. Canadian Journal of Surgery. 2012;**55**(4):264

[40] Scott WJ, Allen MS, Darling G, et al. Video-assisted thoracic surgery versus open lobectomy for lung cancer: A secondary analysis of data from the American College of Surgery Oncology Group Z0030 randomized clinical trial. The Journal of Thoracic and Cardiovascular Surgery. 2010;**139**:976

[41] Burton BN, Khoche S, A'Court AM, et al. Perioperative risk factors associated with postoperative unplanned intubation after lung resection. Journal of Cardiothoracic and Vascular Anesthesia. 2018;**32**:1739

[42] Onaitis M, D'Amico ZY, et al. Risk factors for atrial fibrillation after lung cancer surgery: Analysis of the Society of Thoracic Surgeons general thoracic surgery database. Annals of Thoracic Surgery. 2010;**90**:368

[43] Frendl G, Sodickson AC, Chung MK, et al. 2014 AATS guidelines for the prevention and management of perioperative atrial fibrillation and flutter for thoracic surgical procedures. Executive summary. Journal of Thoracic Cardiovascular Surgery. 2014;**148**:772

[44] Udelsman BV, Soni M, Madariaga ML, et al. Incidence, aetiology and outcomes of major postoperative heamorrhage after pulmonary lobectomy. European Journal of Cardio-Thoracic Surgery. 2020;**57**:462